A Loving Approach to Dementia Care

A
Loving
Approach to
Dementia
Care

THIRD EDITION

MAKING MEANINGFUL CONNECTIONS
WHILE CAREGIVING

Laura Wayman

Johns Hopkins University Press
Baltimore

© 2021 Johns Hopkins University Press
All rights reserved. Published 2021
Printed in the United States of America on acid-free paper
2 4 6 8 9 7 5 3 1

Johns Hopkins University Press
2715 North Charles Street
Baltimore, Maryland 21218-4363
www.press.jhu.edu

Library of Congress Cataloging-in-Publication Data

Names: Wayman, Laura, 1955– author.
Title: A loving approach to dementia care : making meaningful connections while caregiving / Laura Wayman.
Description: Third edition. | Baltimore : Johns Hopkins University Press, 2021. | Series: A Johns Hopkins Press health book | Includes bibliographical references and index.
Identifiers: LCCN 2020013527 | ISBN 9781421440064 (paperback) | ISBN 9781421440071 (ebook)
Subjects: LCSH: Dementia—Patients—Care—Popular works. | Alzheimer's disease—Patients—Care—Popular works.
Classification: LCC RC521 .W39 2021 | DDC 616.8/31—dc23
LC record available at https://lccn.loc.gov/2020013527

A catalog record for this book is available from the British Library.

Special discounts are available for bulk purchases of this book. For more information, please contact Special Sales at specialsales@press.jhu.edu.

Johns Hopkins University Press uses environmentally friendly book materials, including recycled text paper that is composed of at least 30 percent post-consumer waste, whenever possible.

CONTENTS

THANKS AND APPRECIATION

I thank my dear husband, Stephen Wayman, for his patience and support (Boy, has he had a lot of it!). He has steadfastly continued to be my pillar of light, my fountain of love, and a constant source of comfort along the second leg, and now third leg of this amazing journey.

To my daughter Alicia, for her contributions as a supporting author and encourager. To my daughter Angie, who was always the long-distance promoter, silently cheering me on from afar. And to all of my family, who have been there for me all along the way.

To those who have continued to support me through the long birthing process (including this third time around!): DanaLyn Brophy, Teri Crocker, Pamela Dallas, Joe Dunham, Dr. Barbara Gillogly, Cindy Gustafson, Jocelyn Kaufenberg, Rob Stewart, and Andrea Campisi, Jay Zimmer, Caroline Allen, Eric Stone, Audra D'Agostino, Gillian Isaacs-George, Sophie Slater, Rachel VanDyke, Clark Wright, Tammy Cahill, Melinda Klick, Maria Xarias, Katie Wayman, Theresa Haleen, Carol Allen, Mayor John Goodwin, Blake and Candace Ellington, as well as my many other dementia-aware champions too numerous to fit on this page. I could not raise dementia awareness worldwide without you.

A very special thanks to Denise Howard, whose expert editing and copywriting made this third edition of the book once again flow and come together with beauty and grace. Her kind words, professionalism, and conviction gave me the strength to make it to this third finish line. She is my dear friend who held my hand and whispered the necessary nurturing encouragement and constructive advice.

I want to express my heartfelt appreciation for the warm and supportive response I have received as a new, as well as a now third edition, author from everyone at Johns Hopkins University Press in readying my work to be presented to the world. From day one, getting communication and guidance from executive editor Jacqueline Wehmueller for the first and second edition, and now for this third go-round, from Joe Rusko and Adelene Jane Medrano, has been an overall positive experience way beyond what "thank you" can express. And the entire JHUP team has worked, and continues to work, tirelessly with me, all the while presenting profound consideration, understanding, and professional commitment. Truly you all are a shining example of the gold standard in customer service, showing Johns Hopkins University Press as the leader and innovator in scholarly publishing worldwide.

To all the caregivers who honored me with their stories, struggles, strength, moments of success, and commitment.

And a very sincere thank-you to the countless people who initiated this whole project by asking me, "Do you have a book?" (and more recently by the question, "When can we read your third edition?").

This book is dedicated to the loving memory of my mother.

A Loving Approach to Dementia Care

CHAPTER ONE

Introduction

Navigating the Journey

Caring for a person who has dementia is a labor of devotion and patience. Sadly, many caregivers selflessly sacrifice their own well-being during the process. In addition, many caregivers, whether they are lay caregivers looking after a loved one at home or professionals working in a clinical setting, do not have the knowledge or training they need to meet the challenges of dementia. That is exactly where successful caregiving breaks down.

Providing care is an important and noble endeavor, but to be able to provide the best possible care, you must also take care of *yourself*. So pause here and ask yourself one simple question: would it be okay with you, the caregiver, if you experienced a lasting sense of relief?

I have asked many caregivers this question.

Not surprisingly, not one has answered "No."

If you are caring for someone with a form of dementia (such as Alzheimer disease) or another cognitive impairment, this book is intended to help lighten your load every day. It is possible to simultaneously provide better care for the person with dementia and for yourself.

Of course, every family and situation is different. You may have been thrust into this caregiving role unexpectedly—without any training or even any encouragement. Perhaps the care is being provided at home, with or without other family or professional in-home support. Or maybe the care is provided in a specialized memory care unit, an assisted living environment, or a skilled nursing facility. Although caregiving is often inspiring and rewarding, it can be very difficult. Caring for someone with a cognitive impairment can be even more difficult than caring for someone with a physical impairment who is fully competent mentally and emotionally. The complications of confusion, forgetfulness, and memory loss, and the behaviors that go along with them, can be traumatic for the person with the disease and for the person providing care. Because of the dementia, neither the persons involved nor the relationship will ever be the same.

Along with the challenges of caring for a person who has a form of dementia, caregivers—especially family members—will experience conflicting emotions. Their feelings may swing from guilt, denial, and distress one moment to empathy, acceptance, and understanding the next. Not every circumstance is happy, positive, or easy. You may only rarely come to a place of acceptance or understanding about this experience, or maybe not at all. You may struggle to find any meaning along the road you are traveling.

During my decades of working with caregivers, I have heard many accounts of what the experience is like—from the sad and hollow to experiences rich in significance. Everyone faces obstacles when caring for a loved one; some of these obstacles come in the form of uncomfortable or painful emotional histories or past unresolved conflicts. Yet with an open mind, you can essentially "feel your way" through the process, taking a more holistic view of your unique dementia care circumstances and challenges. The following popular fable gently illustrates how each person's perception of dementia, however different it may be from someone else's experience, is nevertheless "right."

The Elephant and the Blind Men

Once upon a time, there lived six blind men in a village. One day, the villagers told them, "Hey, there is an elephant in the village today."

They had no idea what an elephant was. They decided, "Even though we would not be able to see it, let us go and feel it." All of them went to the elephant. Every one of them touched the elephant.

"Hey, the elephant is like a pillar," said the first man, who touched the leg of the elephant.

"Oh, no! It is like a rope," said the second man, who touched the tail.

"Oh, no! It is like a thick branch of a tree," said the third man, who touched the elephant's trunk.

"It is like a big hand fan," said the fourth man, who touched the ear.

"It is like a huge wall," said the fifth man, who touched the belly.

"It is like a solid pipe," said the sixth man, who touched the tusk.

The men began to argue about the elephant, and every one of them insisted that he was "right." A wise man was passing by. He stopped and asked them what was the matter.

"We cannot agree on what the elephant is like," they told him.

And the wise man calmly explained: "All of you are right. Each one of you has a different idea because each of you touched a different part of the elephant. So, actually, the elephant has all of those features—everything you all said."

That ended the argument. They all were happy that they all were "right."

Anekantvad, or *The Theory of Manifold Predictions*

I originally read this fable when I was young. At the time, I was amused by the poor blind man who had to feel the tail. Of course, there could be serious implications with that particular anatomical end of an elephant. Years later, I know that as a caregiver, you may feel as if you are living out a more contemporary proverb: "Some days you're the pigeon, and some days you're the statue."

Your loved one (or client or resident, if you are a professional caregiver) may have a variety of challenges that stem from physical, emotional, and behavioral causes. Perhaps the person you are caring for is unable to communicate clearly without crying, due to a brain injury that diminished his or her ability to control sad or painful emotions. You may be caring for a parent who was verbally or even physically abusive to you or who did not make you feel safe and loved as a child. Now you are attempting to develop a new relationship, even though you cannot erase your feelings or memories. As a result of these and many other factors, you are touching only part of the dementia "elephant," able to view only part of the situation that the dementia has inserted into your life.

I have spent many years assisting caregivers just like you. As you read about the diverse experiences that I and others have had working with dementia-challenged adults, their families, and professional caregivers, you will gain more insight into the intriguing world where the adult with dementia exists. You will also develop a new perspective on many of the common obstacles facing care providers and learn to enjoy your loved one or client at a deeper level. This book—and the special techniques described within it—will equip you with the compass you need to navigate this journey successfully.

Caregivers frequently ask for the "right way" to respond to the difficult behaviors they encounter. While there is no one-size-fits-all magic formula, there are many proven techniques to help guide you. My personal studies in this field have included excellent foundational resources, such as *The Validation Breakthrough*, by Naomi Feil; *The 36-Hour Day*, by Nancy L. Mace and Peter V. Rabins; and *The Best Friend's Approach to Alzheimer's Care*, by Virginia Bell and David Troxel.

My vision is to share as much knowledge and insight with you as possible, both from my own experiences and from those of other professional and family caregivers. Each chapter chronicles a real-life story about caregiving. You may very well find yourself relating to these heartwarming accounts. Every story is followed by two sections, "Lessons Learned" and "Perceptions and Approaches," which can empower you and make your situation more manageable. Use these tools to make traveling this frequently arduous trek much less stressful and much more successful.

In the chapters of this book I describe the *affirmative response method of communication*. This communication style is based on the insight that it is impossible to bring adults with dementia "into reality." Instead of attempting to correct the dementia-challenged person's perception of the world, you can learn to affirm your loved one or client's view of reality and to relate to him or her within that framework. As you give affirmative responses to the dementia-challenged person, you will receive the same from him or her in return, confirming that you have successfully made a connection.

The affirmative response method uses simple and valuable techniques to facilitate quality interactions and enhanced emotional connections with the person who has dementia. These interactions and communications reduce the caregiver's stress level. This innovative approach to communicating opens a window into the world where your loved one or client exists. It will increase your awareness of the equally important need for your own care and the vital role you play in the caregiver–care receiver relationship.

As I travel the country supporting, training, and encouraging caregivers on their dementia journey, I continue to learn additional care techniques. To bring the new techniques to readers of this edition, I created "The Dementia-Aware Guide to Caregiving," which appears at the end of the book (after chapter 21). Here you will find brief examples of common challenges, followed by different options for providing loving care in that specific scenario. This feature of the book allows you to spend a few moments thinking through how you might respond in these situations. You may decide to change just one or two things in your caregiving approach—and that may make a big difference right away for you, your loved one, and your relationship.

When you become a caregiver for someone with dementia, whatever its cause, the key is to shift your mindset to becoming more dementia-aware. Doing so will help you to transform your dementia care experience from crisis to comfort. After each opportunity to raise awareness and understanding about how dementia impacts individuals, their families, and their communities, I have been gratified to witness enhanced feelings of hope and comfort for all involved.

My experience, observations, and research over years of working with family and professional caregivers, as well as dementia-challenged adults, have shown me that using the affirmative response method of communication, in combination with the stress-management tools and the fresh dementia-aware insights described in this book, help caregivers experience many more meaningful moments with the person they are caring for. I believe that you *can* allow yourself to experience a lasting sense of relief and that communication and stress management are the crucial ingredients in doing so. I work with family and professional caregivers as a consultant, often assisting with difficult behaviors and developing a care plan. Whenever I use a tried-and-true technique from my program and have a successful outcome, the observing caregiver will ask me something like this: "How did you do that? Mom doesn't respond to me that way." I immediately explain that I am able to enter the situation from an outside perspective, without the limitations of the baggage that develops over many years of a long relationship. My perspective allows me to view more than just the single dimension of the "elephant" that is immediately obvious: the dementia and the undesired behavior. Unlike a frustrated, on-the-verge-of-burning-out caregiver who may project negativity, I am able to come in with a fresh approach, and the person with dementia is more receptive.

This does not mean that only someone from outside of the relationship can achieve the same results. Regardless of the current dynamic between you and your loved one or client, you can enjoy positive results by approaching the situation from a new angle. Repeatedly I have seen the benefits of viewing the "elephant" from a broader perspective while still keeping key principles in mind. The case studies you are about to read will help you develop a new perspective. As you apply the techniques in this book, celebrate even the smallest accomplishments and moments of heartfelt connection.

I wish it were possible for me to spend time with all of my readers and to learn from you. It is my hope that through this book I will enter your home or your professional caregiving setting and work alongside you. You will find valuable information from my own experiences and from those of the hundreds of caregivers with whom I have had the honor of working.

To complement this book, I highly recommend that all caregivers connect with additional resources. The Lone Ranger made quite a name for himself, but caregiving should never be a solo role. Take, for example, the superhero, Superman! He is portrayed as a hero that is seemingly unbeatable and unstoppable in the comic book world and usually spends his time saving everyone throughout the universe, however, there are times when the "Man of Steel" needs help, too. It happens to everyone, even to the most powerful superhero around! Reach out to your community and ask for help from professional care providers, gerontologists, social workers, educators, physicians, nurses, nationwide organizations such as the Alzheimer's Association, senior centers, caregiver resource centers, caregiver support group facilitators, family members, neighbors, and other caregivers who are in similar situations. Every day, special people in these positions teach me something new and helpful.

As you read about the affirming responses and positive action statements practiced by countless lay caregivers and professional care providers, you will, I hope, grant yourself a creative license to develop your own personal care plan—to create resourceful and imaginative methods to provide better care for your loved one or client, and for yourself.

We are now embarking on this journey together, and we will meet many amazing and inspiring people along the way.

CHAPTER TWO

Peggy

The Ultimate Toll

With Alicia Murray

Peggy was a wonderful mother of five, grandmother of fourteen, and wife to her husband, Jack. Over the years, Peggy and Jack had carefully planned for a fun retirement. Their goal was to spend time with the kids and grandkids and travel all over the United States. They had decided years before that they would sell their home at retirement, buy a recreational vehicle, and live the carefree life. And that's what they did, visiting their relatives scattered all over the West and square dancing everywhere they went. After fifteen years in the RV, Peggy sensed that the change to a larger, more stable home was on the horizon. Her large and growing family could not stay with her in the RV, and she needed more space to entertain them.

Also, Jack's health and eyesight had started to decline, and Peggy had to do more of the driving. So Peggy and Jack made the decision to sell their home on wheels. They found a double-wide mobile home in a small town in northeastern Colorado, which they could afford on their limited budget. It had the disadvantage of being located far away from hospitals, doctors, and senior services, but it had the advantage of being next door to their best friends of forty years. They happily settled in.

Three years passed and Peggy started to have conversations with her children about Jack's memory loss and other symptoms of dementia. Some of her friends had been caregivers of spouses with dementia, and she had seen what a hard and stressful job it was. Her daughter offered to help, but Peggy insisted she was okay and would alert her if his condition became unmanageable.

Two weeks after this conversation, disaster struck. When Jack and Peggy sat down to dinner, Peggy suffered a massive heart attack. Jack's reactions to this emergency were slowed by his dementia, which was far more advanced than anyone had realized. By the time the neighbors called 911 and the EMTs arrived from the faraway emergency services, Peggy was already gone.

Lessons Learned

After Peggy's sudden death, the family realized what a high level of care she had been giving Jack twenty-four hours a day, seven days a week, for several years. The common tragedy of sudden caregiver illness or death illustrates why stress management is so important for caregivers. Caring for a person with dementia is described by the National Family Caregivers Association as being three times more work (and stress) than caring for someone with other types of illnesses. It is a long journey, and if caregivers do not take time for themselves, they will not be around to care for the person with dementia.

Peggy's case is a classic example of the devastating effects of caregiver stress. She was not able to paint a precise picture of how much care Jack was receiving (or how much she herself needed) or to ask for help, even though family, neighbors, and friends had continually offered to help over the years. She was just doing what she had always done, believing she could do it alone. It ended up taking her life.

The sheer amount of work caregivers perform can be overwhelming. For the dementia-challenged adult, basic activities of daily living (ADLs) such as bathing, toileting, and dressing become hard to manage. Many caregivers get so involved in helping that they forget how important they are as the caregiver.

In case my message remains unclear, let me say it again: *If you do not take care of yourself, you will not be able to care for your loved one or client.*

When I teach my caregiver training classes, I often ask family caregivers a simple question: "Who is the most important person?" I am frequently amazed to hear silence in the room; caregivers struggle with that question because they always put the dementia-challenged care recipients first. After all, it is their job to take care of their loved ones and clients, not to take care of themselves. Right?

Wrong. Caregivers are often uncomfortable with being aware of how they, themselves, are the key ingredient in the caregiving process! At one of my training sessions on communication and stress management, an attendee brought along his wife. I observed that she was showing early signs of dementia, and during our class I asked that same question, "Who is the most important person?" His wife was the first to answer, as she lovingly pointed to her husband and said, with a smile, "He is!" She knew, even in her dementia, how important her husband was in that caregiver–care recipient relationship. Learn to take care of *you* as well as your loved one. Learn how to manage and cope with stress along the caregiving journey.

Perceptions and Approaches

My years of observations and interactions have taught me that communicating with the dementia-challenged person involves much more than the words coming out of your mouth. Most of the communication comes from tone of voice, facial expression, and body language. Adults with dementia communicate on the basis of emotions.

Many caregivers do not relate the stress that they are feeling to the trying behaviors the dementia-challenged person is exhibiting, when in fact dementia-challenged people are like a mirror of emotions. For example, if you try to rush them with "Hurry up" or "We don't have time," you will experience resistance in the form of slowed responses or a lack of interest in getting ready. If you glare, tap your foot with impatience, approach the person with your arms crossed in front of you, or make frustrated gestures or sounds—such as rolling your eyes or sighing—you are likely to see those signals "mirrored" back at you in behaviors.

If you are stressed, anxious, and fatigued, the person with dementia will sense it but will not be able to understand what is causing your emotions. When you can reduce the stress in your life and begin to exist in a place of serenity, you will see the entire caregiving experience begin to transform. This is another reason it is so important to keep you, the caregiver, in a place of calmness. It is not only for your own benefit (physically and emotionally) but also to help the person for whom you are caring feel safe, secure, and cooperative throughout the caregiving day.

If only I could have reached Peggy before it was too late—but she was my gentle teacher, showing me that selfless caregivers will take on too much, refusing to ask for or accept help. They will try with all their might to keep promises made long ago to their loved ones, such as the marriage promise to love in sickness and in health, even to a point of pushing beyond their own capabilities.

And Peggy's story hits home, right into my own heart. You see, Peggy was my mother and my children's grandmother, our very own family hero. This personal experience has driven my passion for educating all caregivers, both family and professional, in the awareness of caring for themselves, along with providing tips and tools to assist them in effectively caring for memory-challenged adults. My vision is to bring light into the darkness of dementia through support, encouragement, and hope.

CHAPTER THREE

Deborah

A Daughter's Journey

〜 〜 〜

The signs were subtle and appeared only occasionally at first. The devious brain-destroying disease called Alzheimer's crept up unannounced and began stealing my mom a piece at a time. Alzheimer's is a shrewd and cunning enemy, sneaking in and not clearly identifying itself or even declaring a conventional plan of destruction. "Maybe she's just getting old," I told myself when I first started seeing the symptoms. This was my first bout of dementia-denial, convincing myself it was all a passing nuisance and "no big deal." Then, over time, the progressive failing of her abilities, contrasting from what had been typical for her, began to be more visible. Mom started having more and more difficulty keeping up with mealtime conversations, or she would get easily distracted when performing everyday tasks like cleaning up after a dinner, uncharacteristically leaving dirty dishes on the table or forgetting to put away leftovers. Yet, I still found ways to deny the possibility that this was dementia. After all, she still had a pretty good memory.

While she was exhibiting some occasional short-term memory loss, she could still recall crystal clear details from her past. She was often willing and able to perform detailed familiar tasks to completion or engage in conversation like usual. Just when I would feel a sense of ease, I would witness her struggle to recall the right words when talking about an article she had just read in the newspaper or faltering with the fine points and details when she was discussing a thought or idea. In the beginning, Mom would compensate by changing the subject or replacing the elusive thought or word with another. And when I would observe her compensating, I would tell myself she was experiencing an occasional brain interruption—we all have those, right? But then she started having a problem understanding and following even a simple plot or storyline on a television show. Still fueled by denial, my inner voice would say, "She is just tired," or "Perhaps she is having trouble hearing the television—it was her hearing, right?" Back and forth I volleyed my feelings of acceptance that this was short-lived and would be "fixed" by waiting it out. But I was plagued by fear that even more indisputable failings would rear their ugly heads. I would search for solace by convincing myself that my feelings of denial were justified whenever Mom would have her "moments of clarity" and appear to me as her "normal self."

I want to pause for a moment and make it clear that I did not have a sudden profound moment of acceptance that this situation was serious and getting worse. My lack of "dementia-awareness" kept me in this roller-coaster state of perplexity for a very long time. It did not help that Mom's slow decline was spread out over several years, and this lengthy span slowed my own cognizance that this situation went far beyond just "getting old." Her gradual decline kept "fooling me" until the symptoms became unmistakable. Yes, even though I saw my mom struggling to maintain her very being and saw her clearly overwhelmed with even familiar and everyday tasks, I still sought out the emotional safety of my illusory place within denial. About a year into this journey, I had insisted that Mom see her doctor about these early symptoms. I went with her to this initial appointment, and we both received his toned-down diagnosis of "mild cognitive impairment." When we did not hear the dreaded word "Alzheimer's," the news was perceived by both of us as not so bad—certainly no need to panic or worry. After all, "mild cognitive impairment" is not as serious as "Alzheimer's" or "dementia," right?

This "benign" diagnosis also did not push me to be aware of the need to know more in order to make good care decisions from the beginning. I wanted to believe that I could fix her, or change the progression, or stop the decline. I wanted to believe it would go away, she would get better, and that I would not have to go toe to toe with this relentless monster. I continued to lean on the defense mechanism of denial, justifying my feelings again and again whenever Mom would tap into her diminishing cognitive abilities and misstep, or when she would access the portion of her presently unscathed brain function and appear normal. It was in these "normal" moments that I would feel validated that her symptoms were really not that bad, just "mild cognitive impairment" and not the scary "D" word, dementia, at all.

But what was really happening was that I was moving in and out of acceptance and self-deception. So, I just kept "observing," "taking note," and turning my head, attempting to fix it all in my mind. I continued to implement inadequate short-term solutions such as using sticky notes or verbal reminders, and even correcting Mom when she did not get a detail or word right, forgot to take her medication, or did not remember something I had just told her.

Of course, gradually the cruel progression of the dementia took over, and no sticky notes or verbal reminders or corrections or short in-and-out visits could withstand the dementia's devastating impact on her mind. Mom would get very anxious when I would show up at her door, even though I had told her an hour before I was on my way. She would mix up her medications, taking them at the wrong time or not at all. She even stopped taking a shower and changing her clothes regularly. Visit after visit I observed her wearing the same dirty black turtleneck, black sweatpants, and gloves (even inside the house, as she was always complaining of the cold, even in the heat of summer). She was also having more physical difficulties—losing her balance, shuffling and falling often. I would notice bruises and injuries, and when I would ask her about them, she could not explain where they had come from or remember where or when or if she had fallen.

Then late one night I got a call from a neighbor. They had found Mom wandering out in her driveway in her nightgown, obviously in a state of extreme confusion. It was suddenly undeniably clear that she could not be left alone, so I resolved to move in with her.

After that difficult life-changing decision, it became almost impossible to find consolation in ignoring the inevitable or turning the other way. My unrealistic rationalizations—based in desperate denial—could no longer hide the horrible reality that this was dementia—progressive and permanent loss of her vital brain functions. Mom's increasing loss of ability made me sit up and take notice full time now. Yet my newfound awareness only unearthed the fact that it was also challenging and expensive to find help. I soon discovered that no one had yet developed a simple test for Alzheimer's or for most of the other hundred-plus causes of dementia. Although there was ongoing research and new technology allowing for more detailed brain imaging, these tests still only gave clues and allowed for better educated guesses about the causes of brain function loss. Mom's primary care doctor did not feel comfortable diagnosing the cause as Alzheimer disease or another possible cause of her dementia symptoms without enough evidence from more comprehensive testing, so we were referred to a neurologist who specialized in dementia. In my quest to become more "dementia-aware," I learned that there is no one simple test to tell you if your loved one has it or not. Though medical professionals could gather clues from symptoms and draw reasonable conclusions from them, there was no easy, precise, or clear-cut path to a diagnosis.

When Mom's symptoms became so challenging she could no longer manage her memory loss without constant supervision and care, then and only then did I accept the true and realistic fact that she had permanent and progressive loss of normal brain function—in other words, dementia! This is when I came out from under the umbrella of denial and knew what really counted. It did not matter so much about what the diagnosis was or the cause of her growing list of dementia symptoms; it mattered more to me how well she could function and how my role was now one of dealing directly with what I saw, taking action, and developing an effective care plan. It was crucial that this plan be grounded in care strategies such as: staying in the moment with her; providing her with appropriate emotional, personal, and physical care; keeping her safe; and managing her complicated symptoms and behaviors.

I now look back and realize that had I been "dementia-aware" from the beginning, I could have saved myself and, more importantly, my mom, much aggravation and anxiety on this journey. How I wish I had known then what I have learned since.

Lessons Learned

It is human to deny what we find unpleasant or frightening. But when denial prevents us from seeing facts and facing their implications, it will not help us or our loved ones. In most countries, there is a lack of awareness and understanding of dementia, resulting in stigma and barriers to diagnosis and care, both of which negatively impact caregivers, families, and societies—physically, psychologically, and economically. Dementia is overwhelming not only for the people who have it, but also for their caregivers, family members, and local communities.

Because nobody wants a loved one to have dementia, caregivers are vulnerable to a particular kind of denial. I call it "dementia-denial," and it is based in both self-defense and self-protection. Ultimately, denial will make the dementia care journey much more treacherous. Dementia-denial causes a caregiver to go along with the person's insistence that he or she is "fine" or "normal." Caregivers in dementia-denial often continue to let loved ones make risky decisions, such as driving a car or overseeing finances far longer than is safe, and neglect to develop a legal and financial plan to step in as the decision-maker. Dementia-denial is a hindrance to putting systems in place to protect against many kinds of potentially dangerous abnormal behaviors, allowing them to continue unchecked until someone is injured.

The antidote for "dementia-denial" is to become "dementia-aware." A caregiver who is dementia-aware is one who understands that he or she must seek education about his or her loved one's condition. A dementia-aware caregiver displays a high level of knowledge of the many moving parts of dementia symptoms, the multitude of causes, and tools to adapt and respond. A dementia-aware caregiver gets help in order to make sure that he or she will have sustained energy and resilience during the dementia care marathon. Choosing to operate from a place of acceptance instead of denial is a vital part of being a dementia-aware caregiver.

Perceptions and Approaches

Here's what becoming a dementia-aware caregiver looks like:

• *Dementia-aware caregivers access support from the medical community.* Denying that there are dementia symptoms can delay getting treatment and an appropriate care plan for an individual. Such delays in treatment may allow dangerous declines in health and well-being. This can make dementia more difficult to treat and have consequences on overall quality of life—for both the person with dementia and you, the caregiver. If initial testing only results in a diagnosis of "early dementia" or "mild cognitive impairment," it is not a signal to the caregiver and other family members that everything is okay and no one needs to plan ahead. This is still a serious situation that may and probably will get worse. Neurologists and primary care physicians experienced in dementia need ample time to run tests and assess each individual patient's symptoms. And most of the medications to help with dementia symptoms work best if they are given when the symptoms are exhibited and monitored early on in the dementia journey.

• *Dementia-aware caregivers remain open to continuing education about their loved ones' conditions.* You may have learned a lot about dementia initially, but it is important to stay ahead of the curve and keep learning, as a progressive dementia will continue to alter and diminish your loved one's abilities. Most forms of dementia are progressive, which means every month/day/moment can bring changes. The hard reality is that the definition of "normal" must be continually revised. The higher your level of knowledge early on in the care journey, the more accepting and aware you will be as a caregiver. Maintain realistic expectations that these changes will happen so you can remain fluid and flexible in your care plan and approach.

• *Dementia-aware caregivers consider the bigger picture.* It is not just about your loved one's life. Consider the safety of your loved one and others who might be affected, such as other drivers or pedestrians on the road. While we understand that losing a driver's license is a particularly uncomfortable situation for most people to talk about, it is important to understand that denial has a ripple effect on others.

• *Dementia-aware caregivers continuously reach out to stay supported all along the way.* It is important to be sustained by family, neighbors, friends, and other caregivers through support groups, professionals in the community, and ongoing education. *It takes a village to care for a loved one with dementia.* Once dementia-denial has been alleviated by dementia-awareness, family members and professionals can begin to seek the best avenues available for treatment and care for their loved ones, clients, or residents with dementia.

Dementia-awareness must go well beyond the individual family or professional caregiver, even to those who are not presently on a personal dementia care journey. Millions of Americans are already affected by this disease, and that number is expected to rapidly grow during the coming decades. As a society, we must become more dementia-aware and able to direct caregivers and persons with dementia to appropriate support resources. And that starts by being dementia-aware on an individual level.

Here's what a dementia-aware community looks like:

As the number of dementia cases continues to increase locally, nationwide, and worldwide, there is a growing need for caregivers, healthcare leadership and staff, clergy, local community government, leadership, the general population, and all first responders—firemen and law enforcement—to become "dementia-aware." Specialized training (dementia-awareness) is necessary to cultivate a deeper understanding and clearer recognition of dementia and how it affects those living with or caring for anyone presenting its symptoms. Such training imparts knowledge of appropriate, competent, and sensitive "dementia-aware" care and service, supporting not only those with dementia symptoms but all the local community members, as well as their family and professional care providers.

a. Unfortunately, with Alzheimer's and other forms of dementia, there are no known processes for recovery. The dementia symptoms will increase and the individual will decline in cognitive ability over time. The dementia sufferer can no longer determine their own course of action, or take responsibility for their actions. Community-wide, dementia-aware training must be based in the knowledge that all services are provided with positive reflection and a meaningful understanding of those experiencing dementia symptoms and those who are living with them and caring for them.

b. In an emergency, people with dementia and their caregivers may find themselves uprooted or displaced to alternative living arrangements. Extra care and attention must be made to ensure the health, security, and safety of the individual with any cause of dementia symptoms. Dementia-awareness training has been uniquely developed to better prepare law enforcement and the fire department to understand and proficiently handle the challenges facing their citizens with dementia, and the ripple effect these challenges have on not just the caregiver, but the entire community.

c. Dementia-aware trainings, presented in an easy to understand and practical method, address these individuals' needs and values, with not only an acknowledgment that personal differences exist but also a respect for these differences. In order to be sufficiently prepared for these and many other dementia symptoms and challenges, everyone, across the community, must become "dementia-aware."

d. Diverse senior and "dementia-aware" care resources and options will assist in providing better quality of life, a safe living environment, appropriate supervision and care, while also fostering a sense of hope and optimism for first responders, *all* community members, and leadership, as well as for the beleaguered family care providers and those to whom they provide care.

I recently had the opportunity to raise dementia-awareness for the Cosumnes CSD Fire Department, located in Elk Grove, California. Directly after the four-hour workshop that firemen, policemen, paramedics, and medical personnel had attended, I received this email (one of many excellent examples of how becoming dementia-aware can benefit our first responders as they interact with the many members of their community living with varying levels of brain function loss and dementia symptoms) from two of the grateful participants:

Dear Laura,

The dementia class paid off in no time at all! Eddie (**Eddie Raschein**, Firefighter/Paramedic, **Cosumnes CSD Fire Department**) and I wanted to share with you our experience later in the day after your wonderful presentation.

Eddie was contacted by an Engine crew who was called to a private residence to assist a wife who could not get her husband out of their vehicle. The older gentleman had Dementia in advanced stages. Although pleasant, he would not voluntarily exit the family car to his house. He was conversive, although confused, and at times his words were unrecognizable, but he sure knew what he was saying! The compassionate Captain and crew [were] concerned as to how to assist the wife with the least physical means possible.

Armed with our new skills, away we flew! Your pearls of dementia-aware wisdom for how to observe and approach the person with dementia was fresh in our heads, but the first thing Eddie said was "How are you doing?" as soon as we got there! (oops, no questions!) From there, we quietly observed the patient and his situation. He was a bilateral amputee and would require assistance with transfer from the car to the wheelchair. During the observation, it was clear the family pet dog was a focus of love for this gentleman. After practicing some affirmation statements with him, I said "It's dinner time. The dog needs to eat. Let's take the dog into the house and feed him." This seemed to resonate with him. He stated back "I don't have any money and can't go into the house." Again, a positive affirmation "We don't need any money today." That was then his focus . . . time to feed the dog. In the house.

With tender patience and empathy, the gentleman transferred himself to his awaiting wheelchair. Pushed by wonderful paramedics, he and the dog entered the house under his own will. His wife was the EXACT selfless caregiver you described in your stories. She herself had a not too old scar peeking out from her summer top neckline, indicating recent major heart surgery. The new sense of concern was present on our minds.

We did not part without leaving this superhero of a wife with some suggestions for support, including your website. Additionally, Eddie and I were able to debrief with the crew in a very quick synopsis of the condition of dementia, the process and communication strategies you had taught us only hours before. We are thankful to have some better direction on how to assist this couple.

We look forward to offering this course in the future to all of the healthcare providers at CFD. We will continue to communicate with you and plan the next course of action. Warmly,

Juliet Carrington, RN CADS, EMS Performance and
    Development Coordinator
Certified Ambulance Documentation Specialist,
    Designated Infection Control Officer
Cosumnes Fire Department, Elk Grove, CA

Here are some additional, quality-assured dementia-awareness raising community resources who are promoting ways of more successfully living with dementia in communities around the world:

- Dementia Partnerships, Sharing Knowledge and Learning Across the Well Pathway for Dementia: https://dementiapart nerships.com/resource/dementia-awareness-resource-pack/.
- Alzheimer's Europe, Switzerland 2013: National policies covering the care and support of people with dementia and their carers:
  https://www.healthcheck.nhs.uk/increasing-dementia -awareness-training-resource/#1;
  https://www.alzheimer-europe.org/Policy-in-Practice2 /Country-comparisons/2013-National-policies-covering-the -care-and-support-of-people-with-dementia-and-their-carers /Switzerland.

There is good news in that there *is* growing recognition of the importance, across the United States and around the world, for caregivers; healthcare leadership/staff; clergy; local community government; leadership and the general population; all first responders; firemen; and law enforcement to become dementia-aware.

That is why I am so excited that the town of Colma, California, decided to make the commitment to become a "Dementia-Aware Safe Space." After speaking about the importance of this effort to the city council, it was so gratifying that the council members were receptive to it. In fact, they helped to establish a declaration in order to urge all of the various businesses, first responders, leadership, community members, and organizations in the town to complete my series of trainings and workshops in order to benefit the community, as a whole, in becoming dementia-aware. It is such an honor that I was able to designate the entire town and place a "Dementia-Aware Safe Space" sticker on the wall of Colma Town Hall (https://www.laurawayman .com/blog/town-of-colma-becomes-a-certified-dementia-aware-safe -space).

I know there are many more of these opportunities to come as we unite in dementia-awareness, stamping out individual and community-wide dementia-denial, and look to find more and better ways to support those living with dementia symptoms and their caregivers.

Denial from the viewpoint of a caregiver is an entirely different experience than denial from the perspective of the person who has dementia. In the next chapter, Charles's story provides insight into why the person with dementia is also often challenged by denial and how you can navigate this dynamic as a caregiver.

CHAPTER FOUR

Charles

There Is Nothing Wrong with Me

My father, Charles, is a perfect case study and example of the initial acceptance of a dementia diagnosis followed by the relentless change to an apparent dementia-denial of the disease as it progressed.

Charles himself initiated the visit to his primary care physician that resulted in his diagnosis. On his own, he had become increasingly aware of the insidious dementia signs and symptoms before I had even noticed them. At the doctor's appointment, my father was able to discuss with his physician how he was experiencing some sleep difficulties, slowed movements and slight tremors, as well as decline in his cognitive function and ability to process information that had always come so easily to him in the past. Sadly, it turned out to be early-stage Lewy body disease. At that time, he accepted the doctor's verdict with poise. My father and I talked about it, researched it, and made plans together about what we would do. We decided to make the most of the time we had left before the disease started taking over his mind and abilities. By making accommodations for the short-term memory loss and other budding symptoms, we managed to enjoy a few years spending precious time and making special memories—doing all those things we had put off before we received the dreadful diagnosis.

The progression was mercifully slow but painfully steady, especially at the beginning. But over time, the disease began to assume control of his life. His personality changed entirely. If I even brought up the idea of visiting a doctor for any reason, he would become furious. I did not understand what was happening, why my father was changing before my eyes. I had to accept the heart-wrenching reality that this was no longer the father I once knew. The ever-present smile and loving disposition were all but completely gone. The gentle, patient man who for fifty-six years had never had an ill-tempered word for me now frequently exploded with irrational, angry outbursts and uncharacteristic fits of impatience.

It was in the final part of his dementia journey that he became completely unaware of how debilitated he had become. He could no longer remember or process that he had been given the diagnosis early on, or that at one time he had even gracefully accepted the fact. At this point, he had full-blown dementia-denial of his own illness. But this went beyond the normal type of denial so many people experience when facing difficult circumstances, such as the denial I had as a caregiver. Instead, my father had a different kind of denial known as *anosognosia*—literally a lack of knowledge of disease. I later learned that anosognosia [an-o´so-no´zhah] has long been recognized in people with strokes, brain tumors, Alzheimer's, Lewy body, and Huntington's disease, as well as many of the other causes of dementia symptoms. Although this dementia-denial may at first appear to be similar to the denial the caregiver is experiencing, anosognosia is not the same and is far more challenging. Unfortunately, there is no antidote for anosognosia, as there is no way to challenge it with dementia-awareness.

As his son, I was forced to watch my father fade away a piece at a time without having any way to stop it, change it, fix it, or console him by sharing what was happening. Any mention of dementia, Lewy body disease, the decline in his health and abilities, or his progressing care needs would send my father into a rage: "There is nothing wrong with me!" His resistance to my care efforts was nothing short of intense, often with a pinch of paranoia and a handful of spitefulness thrown into the mix. Any attempt on my part to make him understand that he had changed and needed to accept new limits was an exercise in frustration for both of us. It was simply much more successful if, as his primary caregiver, I made all decisions related to his care without discussing them with him or asking for his input or opinion.

On a very basic level, I came to realize my father's "thinker" was broken and that the more I did the "thinking" for him, the kinder and more supportive I remained in his eyes. This all felt weird and crazy, and so contrary to how I had identified my part in this father-son relationship, yet I found that when I changed my communication approach and shared less information concerning his condition and necessary care decisions, he appeared calmer and more at peace. When I finally recognized that he simply "did not know what he did not know" and I accepted that I must do all the "knowing" for him about his care, our dementia journey became less tumultuous, and we were able to experience many more meaningful moments together.

Lessons Learned

In some cases, people with dementia will experience precisely the same kind of dementia-denial their caregivers exhibit, namely that understandable emotional desire to convince ourselves that everything is fine. However, anosognosia is an entirely different problem. While anosognosia is still difficult to define, researchers know it results from physical, anatomical changes or damage to the part of the brain that affects perception of one's own illness. As a neurological impairment, it is common following brain injuries or diseases. For instance, people with a disease or illness causing dementia may display anosognosia and insist they do not have a problem. Naturally, the family member or professional caregiver who has to deal with this problem can become exasperated.

To make the situation even more challenging, anosognosia may be complete or selective, in the latter case only revealing itself in certain situations that trigger the person's dementia-denial, such as when he or she becomes frustrated trying to perform simple daily tasks. The person diagnosed with any form of dementia may be entirely unaware of his or her impairment, or react with anger and defensiveness if confronted about the illness. This makes it difficult to diagnose anosognosia and tough to differentiate it from common dementia-denial. But whether your loved one is in simple denial of his or her dementia or has anosognosia, the most effective caregiving strategy is one of acceptance and empathy toward the symptoms and subsequent behaviors, rather than endlessly trying (and failing) to make the person with dementia understand.

Much more than denial, anosognosia is a far-reaching lack of awareness of impairment—most people do not even know they are ill—and it affects up to 81 percent of people with Alzheimer disease, the leading cause of dementia. After strokes, some studies show up to 77 percent of people suffer with anosognosia. And just like any and all causes and symptoms of dementia, this lack of awareness affects each person differently.

Anosognosia with dementia shows no favoritism with regard to occupation, gender, ethnicity, education, or financial status, as evidenced in the life of President Woodrow Wilson and his personal dementia journey. In 1919, toward the end of his second term, President Wilson suffered a stroke. Following his stroke, the notable feature of the president's behavior was his denial of his incapacity. Denial of illness is a common sequel to the type of brain injury received by President Wilson. In this condition, the patient denies or appears unaware of such physical deficits as paralysis or blindness, as well as loss of other brain functions. To casual observers, anosognosic patients may appear normal and even bright and witty. When not talking about their disability, they can be quite rational, and tests of their intelligence may show no deficit. In President Wilson's case, his anosognosia prevented him from getting the care he needed after his stroke.

Wilson described himself as "lame" and referred to his cane as his "third leg," but otherwise he considered himself perfectly fit to be president. There was even talk of a third term. Yet his close associates noticed a change in his personality and abilities. He became increasingly suspicious, even paranoid, without having the dimmest awareness of the fact that he was perhaps becoming a different person from who he once was. Stockton Axson, his brother-in-law from his first marriage, wrote that President Wilson "would be seized with what, to a normal person, would seem to be inexplicable outbursts of emotion. He was furious at anyone who suggested that he had physical and mental problems, and the last months of his presidency became a graveyard of fired associates."

To explain this type of dementia-denial another way, "Our right brain is wired to detect anomalies and new information and incorporate these into our sense of reality," according to neuroscientist Dr. V. S. Ramachandran, in the *New York Times*. When something happens to damage that part of the brain—such as a stroke, Alzheimer's, or many of the other causes of dementia—then "the left brain seeks to maintain continuity of belief, using denial, rationalization, confabulation and other tricks to keep one's mental model of the world intact."

If you are concerned that your loved one, client, or resident might have dementia complicated by anosognosia, here are some signs to look for:

- Not keeping up with regular daily tasks or personal hygiene.
- Having difficulty managing money or bills.
- Being more spontaneous or less inhibited in conversation without concern for his or her own behavior.
- Becoming angry when confronted with forgetfulness, lack of self-care, poor decision-making, or many other dementia symptoms.
- Confabulating: making up answers that the person believes are true, though sometimes the details may be imaginary, may pertain to something that happened in the past, or even be based on something he or she read or heard elsewhere.

Perceptions and Approaches

Dealing with dementia-denial on the part of the person with dementia is a trying situation for caregivers, who are endeavoring to help someone who essentially does not and cannot acknowledge he or she is ill. People with dementia and anosognosia exhibit obvious difficulties with routine tasks, judgment, and executive thinking skills, yet they often insist they do not need help, even to the point of refusing medical evaluation or treatment, as well as much-needed nonmedical assistance and emotional support.

For caregivers, successfully overcoming dementia-denial involves the ability to learn a new perception and deeper understanding of dementia, and then take that knowledge to develop a care approach that works. People with dementia and anosognosia, however, cannot become dementia-aware, as they will become progressively more incapable of recognizing they have any dementia symptoms, even when their symptoms are very obvious to those who are caring for them. Unlike with caregiver dementia-denial, there is no remedy for the form of denial exhibited by someone with anosognosia.

It is a scary thought to consider. What if you were ill, suffering from dementia, and did not know it? And there was no way to make you understand the complexity of it all? How would your loved ones or treatment providers give you appropriate care if you continued to refuse their well-intentioned and necessary help? This is precisely what many caregivers experience as the person whom they are assisting continues to resist critical support on many different levels. This often leaves the caregiver with the responsibility of providing and accessing appropriate help—needing to make difficult decisions without having buy-in from the one who desperately needs increasing levels of care.

For example, many anguished family caregivers have contacted me about how and when to take away the car keys, while their loved one with dementia is still certain he or she can safely operate an automobile. Another common question concerns when it is time to access out-of-home care. People with dementia and anosognosia will dig in their heels and wholly believe they can stay independent in their own homes and safely care for themselves, even when all the evidence strongly suggests otherwise. Answering these questions and determining the "right time" can be excruciating for the primary caregiver and is another reason why dementia care is such a stressful role. In these situations, you, the caregiver, must cease basing essential care decisions upon what you believe your loved one wants—instead, you must move to the logical response of decisions based on what he or she needs at the time, accessing the care and assistance that will keep your loved one, and everyone around your loved one, safe. Going against your loved one's wishes is seldom the path of least resistance—

on the contrary, it is almost always the path of greatest opposition—and it is an exhausting uphill segment of the dementia journey. But if your loved one has both dementia and dementia-denial—especially denial in the form of anosognosia—it is essential that you take charge of his or her affairs.

Here are five things to keep in mind when caring for someone with dementia symptoms and anosognosia:

1. *Use positive action statements in your communication.* Be gentle, encouraging, and empathetic about necessary tasks. Avoid asking too many questions or giving too many options. Questions can be distressing at the best of times and can put pressure on people. Questions, reasoning, and multiple options become too much information for the person with dementia to process. KEEP IT SIMPLE!

• *Break down activities into a series of steps.* This will help to make many tasks much more manageable. Encourage your loved one to do what they can, gently remind them of steps they tend to forget, and assist with steps they are no longer able to accomplish on their own. Using visual cues, such as showing them with your hand where to place the dinner plate, can be very helpful. Instead of asking "Are you hungry, would you like to eat some lunch?" Change the question into a simple and easily processed positive action statement such as: "Come with me, let's have some lunch together."

• *I like to call this playing "Dementia Jeopardy!"* In other words, give the person with dementia the answer without expecting them to understand or have to respond to the question. Someone with a healthy working brain enjoys considering questions and options and coming up with appropriate responses, they can do this on "autopilot." In people with dementia, when there is loss of brain function in the area that processes questions, options, and decision-making, this will inevitably cause frustration and anxiety for the person when that processing ability is no longer there.

2. *Spend time with no pressure, no agenda, no judgment, and no expectations.* Allow the person to be whoever he or she is right now. Downsize any responsibilities that are unnecessary. Often the answer is a professional in-home caregiver, adult day care, or a memory care com-

munity that is trained in dementia care. It takes a village to care for someone with dementia, so build your village of care professionals, family, friends, and local community members. Remember, you cannot stop, change, or cure the dementia symptoms—you can only help to manage them.

• *Keep in mind* individuals with dementia symptoms often feel confused, anxious, and unsure of themselves, and expectations of them taking part in a normal exchange of dialogue or completing even simple tasks can contribute to even more of these feelings. Further, they often get reality confused and may recall things that never really occurred.

• *Avoid trying to convince them they are wrong.* Stay focused on the feelings they are demonstrating (which are real) and respond with verbal and physical expressions of comfort, support, and reassurance, rather than correcting or reasoning with them. Sometimes just simply being present, holding hands, touching, hugging, and praise will help the person to connect and respond when words, instructions, or a lengthy discussion fail. And because it is necessary to practice this type of care approach and communication twenty-four hours a day, be sure and carve out respite time for yourself. Access help from dementia-aware professionals, family members, friends, and neighbors to give you a break on a regular basis.

3. *Avoid fact- and reason-based discussions with the person who has dementia symptoms and anosognosia* about his or her medical condition or changing care needs. The more you, the caregiver, become dementia-aware, the more you will see that your loved one's comments, behaviors, and changes are an expected part of the disease process and out of his or her control, helping you to better plan and accept what is yet to come. When voicing concerns, stay calm, confident, patient, and present in the moment. Articulate your thoughts in a simple and positive light. Practice communication that excludes discussion about what abilities he or she has lost, all the while increasing the focus and attention on what abilities still remain.

• *Dementia causes such a devastating loss in so many areas*—not just the loss of brain function and abilities in the individual with the dementia symptoms, but also loss of the previous relationship with the caregiver. It becomes very difficult not to expect communication and rapport between them to remain the same. This is often where the caregiver is most challenged, they continue to want to share information as they did before, which ends up causing more anxiety and frustration for both of them. It is necessary to only share the information the person with dementia can process and manage, knowing they cannot do so in the same way they did in the past.

• *Often there is little or no understanding of the extent of care that the person with dementia symptoms is requiring at any given time.* When it comes to accessing appropriate care, the caregiver feels so disheartened when they cannot get their loved one to accept or buy into the overall care plan.

• *A dementia-aware caregiver understands they must make care decisions with the intent of knowing what is best for them both, without having the opportunity to make them any longer as a team.* For example, instead of saying, "We have a caregiver coming to the home to take care of you," try; "I am having a helper come and assist *me* with some household chores so that we can have more time to spend together."

4. *Allow people with dementia the dignity of experiencing whatever emotions they are feeling at the time,* with an understanding that these feelings are real to them, even if they are difficult for you to understand. Although people with dementia may seem distant or confused at times, their emotions and feelings remain. When interacting with people who have dementia, hold their hands, give them a hug. Show them patience, compassion, and care. Attempting to correct or reason with a person who has anosognosia will only result in resistance—a test of frustration for both of you that can generate further feelings of anxiety, even accelerating to more extreme challenging behaviors, such as combativeness and aggression.

• *We have been taught to try to change, fix, or stop what people are feeling.* It is often a new skill to learn to accept and join adults and allow them to stay in their feelings. The more we learn to empathize and join the person with dementia symptoms, the more meaningful moments you will experience with them.

• *If the person with dementia symptoms becomes upset, join and agree with them in their feelings.* For example, propose that they help you with a task or suggest that you both take a walk together. It is important to connect with the person on a feeling level, before you take positive action. You might say, "I see you're feeling sad. Let's go get something to eat."

• *Think of how you might react to someone with a healthy and fully functioning brain who is expressing fear and anxiety.* Perhaps they had a nightmare and woke up screaming and crying. How would you respond? You would probably comfort them by explaining that they were okay and safe, that it was just a dream. Then their brain could go to work and process your words and decide if this made sense, and probably begin to feel better. You have succeeded in changing how they are feeling with your reasoning and this whole back and forth process works more successfully when they are able to "think your reasoning through."

• *Now consider how the person with dementia symptoms, who is no longer able to "think your reasoning through," might feel* if they could indeed hear your comforting words but they did not make sense of what you were saying, so they continued to feel even more fear and anxiety. Then it would be necessary to confirm their feelings (join and agree) so that they can trust you and allow you to join them wherever they are in their dementia-altered reality. They probably are having difficulty processing the difference between the reality when awake and the dreams when they were sleeping; it all feels the same to them. For example, in order to join them start off with an affirmative statement such as, "I see you are really frightened. I feel scared sometimes too. However, when I am near you like this, I feel much safer. Let's go have some tea and take it easy."

Once again, actions speak louder than words and being present, holding hands, touching, hugging, and praise will help the person to connect and respond when just words, instructions, or a lengthy discussion will fail.

5. *Be sure you remember to take care of yourself.* Caregivers often feel obligated to sacrifice themselves for the sake of the person for whom they are caring. As a result of neglecting to care for themselves, care-

givers frequently become burned out and resentful, especially if other family members do not share the burden. Holding regular family meetings and keeping open communication can help clear the air before things reach a breaking point. It is essential to everyone's well-being that you remain in good health and can balance your care responsibilities with your own needs.

• *A person with dementia symptoms needs more and more support and care, but on the other side of the coin, so do the family members and professional caregivers who are caring for them.* It is disheartening to discover that 35 percent of those caring for someone with Alzheimer's, or another form of dementia, say their health has gotten worse because of their duties. It takes a special kind of understanding of its process to effectively care for those suffering from this unforgiving disease. Specialized training (dementia-awareness) is necessary to cultivate a deeper understanding and clearer recognition of dementia and how it affects those living with or caring for anyone presenting its symptoms. The training covers appropriate, competent, and sensitive dementia-aware care and service. This supports not only those with dementia symptoms but anyone who is currently managing someone with the disease.

As you continue to read this book, you will become more and more dementia-aware, helping to sustain you through the many obstacles you will encounter on the road ahead. Whether you are a family caregiver, a professional caregiver, or an individual who wishes to help build a more dementia-aware world, keep in mind that the more you know about the many layers of dementia, the better you will be able not only to navigate your own dementia care journey, but to help others on their personal journeys as well.

CHAPTER FIVE

Frances

What Is Dementia?

Frances walked by with short, scuffling steps. Her body was stooped over; she looked down, not ahead. She seemed unaware of me as she passed, just inches away. She wore a distant look on her weather-worn face and a blank stare in her glazed eyes, but I knew she was aware of my presence. So I said her name.

She paused, lifted her head, and answered, "Yes?"

I said, "Frances, it almost looks as if you are in the middle of a dream and sleepwalking."

Suddenly aware and alert, she looked me in the eye and said, "Absolutely!" Then she slowly turned, her eyes and face as empty as before, and shuffled away.

I had spent several hours with Frances over the previous few weeks and had become aware that she often looked like a sleepwalker, not thoroughly in the same awake existence as I was, but still able to converse or relate to me in my reality for spurts of time. Frances was in the advanced stages of Alzheimer disease and was being assisted lovingly by her only son, who had quit his job to care for her full time.

Her son had contacted me to help him manage some of her challenging behaviors, including her repetitive daily routine and her restlessness during the late evening into nighttime, a phenomenon commonly called sundowning.

Frances slept only two to three hours at night, and during the day she was agitated and restless. She busied herself by taking all of the cups, bowls, and glasses out of the kitchen cabinets, filling them with warm water, and then placing them on the counters, table, and even on the floor. She would then involve herself with her other routine of taking everything out of her closet, spreading clothes and shoes on her bed and on the floor, often taking everything off the hangers and making piles. She never sat down. To get her to eat, her son placed finger foods on a plate on the corner of the table, since she would only eat on the go.

I was curious about Frances's profession before her retirement, and I was fascinated to learn that she had been a baker. For the majority of her life, her daily routine had begun long before sunrise when she would start the yeast processing in warm water. In addition to working as a baker, she had managed a large acreage property. Her son told me about his fond memories of her quick, long strides as she gardened, mowed, picked, and watered to keep her treasured land in tip-top shape.

She had always been busy, busy, busy—driven by her parents' sayings, such as, "The devil finds work for idle hands!" My initial observation was that although the son was coping with her care, he was showing many signs of extreme stress. He was exhausted from the constant interruptions at night and lack of sleep.

My first suggestion was for him to seek out and use regular in-home care and respite. He needed to take time to rest and sleep without his mom continually interrupting him. He also needed time for himself, away from his caregiving responsibilities, to do things he enjoyed. And because knowledge is empowering, he needed to carve out time to get specialized information about dementia and learn more about his mom's illness. With a better understanding of dementia and the behaviors it may cause, the son could customize Frances's care to take into account her distinctive history and needs.

Lessons Learned

The word *dementia* comes from the Latin *dis*, meaning "away from," and *mens*, meaning "mind." It describes a state of being away from your mind or existing in this world while being away from your previous life. Like sleepwalking.

What Is Dementia?

Dementia is not a specific disease. It's an overall term that describes a group of symptoms associated with a decline in thinking skills severe enough to reduce a person's ability to perform everyday activities. What is behind these dementia symptoms? Our brains are always trying to make sense of things, to impose order on all the information we are continuously taking in. But when an individual has dementia symptoms, whole experiences are constantly being lost, making it difficult for the brain to get its bearings. In plain language, the essential parts of the brain that we access and utilize in order to understand the world around us—every piece of data we receive, process, and put to use to do anything—is now broken, and with most causes of dementia, it will continue to be even more broken. The way I like to describe it is that the person presenting dementia symptoms has a "broken thinker" and to become "dementia-aware" is to learn to "think" for them.

Dementia in its various manifestations (for example, issues with cognition, behavior, mood, psychological state, muscle memory, etc.) is a list of *symptoms*, very much like a cough or a fever are common symptoms of the flu. If you have a cough, it does not necessarily mean you have lung cancer, and if you have dementia, it does not necessarily mean the cause of your dementia symptoms is Alzheimer disease. The cough could be a symptom of respiratory influenza, and dementia could be one of several symptoms caused by a stroke, for example. Dementia is often confused with Alzheimer's. But Alzheimer's is a disease (a cause), and the various manifestations of dementia are symptoms, either of the leading cause of dementia—Alzheimer disease—or of another disease or disorder or even exposure to a toxin. If you had a medical exam and the doctor gave you the dreaded news that you were suffering from dementia, the next question you would need to ask is, "What is causing these dementia symptoms?" There are many different causes that could be the possible answer to this question!

As explained by the Alzheimer's Association, "Dementia is not a specific disease. It's an overall term that describes a wide range of symptoms associated with a decline in memory or other thinking skills severe enough to reduce a person's ability." For example, an exposure to anesthesia increases the risk of having dementia symptoms, although anesthesia-induced dementia symptoms are usually temporary. Chemical or other exposure is often misdiagnosed or overlooked as a cause of dementia symptoms. According to the Investigative Clinical Amyloid Research in Alzheimer's (ICARA), the medications or substances that may cause dementia symptoms include the following:

- alcohol
- amphetamines
- atropine (a drug used in anesthesia)
- barbiturates
- bromides (an ingredient in some medications)
- certain anti-Parkinsonian drugs
- certain antispasmodics
- certain tranquilizers
- manganese poisoning
- cocaine (including "crack" cocaine)
- cortisone
- digitalis
- illicit drugs
- lead poisoning
- lithium
- mercury poisoning

Drug interactions and drug withdrawal can also cause dementia symptoms, although it is usually temporary.

In addition, there is a difference between dementia and delirium. Although the symptoms of dementia and delirium are similar, the causes and definitions are not. Dementia is defined as an irreversible state of cognitive impairment and short-term memory loss caused by organic brain disease—most commonly Alzheimer disease or multiple cerebral infarcts (strokes). Delirium, on the other hand, is a state of cognitive impairment, clouding of consciousness, and confusion that improves when the cause is addressed.

Delirium is characterized by a sudden onset of confusion. Symptoms of delirium occur rapidly—not over a long period of time, as happens with dementia. According to the *Merck Manual for Healthcare Professionals*, the most common causes of delirium are

- certain medications—particularly anticholinergics, psychoactive drugs, and opioids
- dehydration
- infection (such as urinary tract infections)

There are some circumstances that can cause people to develop dementia-like symptoms. Depression, dehydration, malnutrition, hospitalization from a severe injury or fall—all can cause a person to behave abnormally. I advise many caregivers to get a thorough medical workup for their loved ones or clients to rule out these other causes of dementia symptoms or delirium. Unfortunately, in contrast to delirium, dementia is a long-term, generally irreversible condition. The most common cause of dementia is Alzheimer disease, between 60 and 80 percent of people with dementia have Alzheimer disease. There are, however, many other causes of dementia, including stroke, Lewy body disease, Parkinson's disease, and head trauma. Many people have a dual diagnosis, with two or more causes, such as Parkinson's and Alzheimer's, or a stroke and Alzheimer's.

People with dementia symptoms may have any of these problems and other problems, as well:

- confusion
- disorientation
- repetitive behaviors
- problems with tracking or processing information
- spatial difficulties, such as having a limited view of physical surroundings, struggles with balance, coordination, and depth perception
- anxiety

- fear
- paranoia

Nearly everyone with dementia has progressive short-term memory loss. The dementia-challenged person may shuffle and be slightly off-balance or have problems with depth perception.

Dementia frequently brings about impaired judgment and a loss of inhibitions, causing individuals to exhibit behaviors that may appear odd and may be out of character for them. In addition, people with dementia may have difficulty making decisions. The person's ability to be organized and to do multiple tasks simultaneously may become limited. Many people with dementia choose not to participate in their usual activities if there is too much outside stimuli.

Do any of these behaviors and problems sound familiar to you as you think about your loved one?

Perceptions and Approaches

As a helpful visualization for understanding the progressive loss of normal brain function, imagine that a healthy human brain is like a block of solid sharp cheddar cheese. In contrast, the brain of a person with dementia looks like a large, traditional wedge of Swiss cheese, with holes spread throughout it. And in the center of that sizeable wedge of perforated Swiss cheese is a hungry rat. The rat in the cheese is the root cause—or source—of the progressive and permanent loss of normal brain function resulting in the growing list of dementia symptoms. In this example, we will name (or diagnose) this rat as Mr. Alzheimer's (a.k.a. the progressive cause of the loss of normal brain function presented as many possible dementia symptoms). Mr. Alzheimer's, in this example, comes in the form of Alzheimer disease—the leading cause of dementia—yet could come in any of the more than one hundred causes of dementia, such as Parkinson's disease, Lewy body disease, Huntington's disease, AIDS, or alcoholism. Regardless, the rat is busily eating away at the block of priceless "cheese" (memory, cognitive function, and personality).

At this time, we do not know how Mr. Alzheimer's (or most of the other one hundred plus causes of normal brain function loss) initially makes his home in the brain. Unfortunately, we also do not have any way to get the rat out, halt, or even slow the damage he causes. And the rat continues running around to all different sections of the brain, nibbling away at the cheese and leaving ever larger holes. Mr. Alzheimer's path of destruction is up to his unique discretion—he may choose to steadily move about and then show bursts of energy and quickly change his course, exposing faster and more abrupt declines in the person's abilities. Or the rat may mosey about, instigating a long and mysterious path of deterioration over many months and years. When working with clients and families, I refer to this phenomenon as the "cheese and holes." Sometimes you may enjoy a day of clarity with your loved one, when he or she is "all there"—that is when you have hit the cheese. And on another day, your loved one may be confused, agitated, or even vacant—you have hit a hole in the cheese.

Being a dementia-aware caregiver involves accepting the unfortunate fact that when the effects of permanent, progressive loss of normal brain function are readily observable, there is no way to stop, alter, or fix the escalating dementia symptoms. Instead, the caregiver needs to implement a realistic care approach, with the understanding that you can only do your best to manage the changes. It is critical for a dementia-aware caregiver to stay fluid and flexible, as the strategies for managing the symptoms will shift in the blink of an eye—or in the next greedy bite of cheese.

I want to help you develop the ability to take hold of and cherish every possible connection with the "cheese" that remains—for as long as you can.

Easier said than done, considering the difficulties of caregiving. Your day must be filled with patience, empathy, and efforts to maintain your loved one's dignity. At the same time, you must manage all the day-to-day activities necessary to feed, clothe, bathe, and nurture the person in your care.

Frances was suffering from the short-term memory loss typical of dementia. Along with the memory loss, Frances may also have been experiencing Capgras syndrome. A person with Capgras syndrome, also known as Capgras delusion, believes that people close to her have been replaced by duplicates. The person with Capgras may doubt her own identity and question whether she, in whole or in part, has been replaced by an impostor. This syndrome is more prevalent in women than in men.

Although the syndrome is most common among people with schizophrenia, it can also occur as a result of a severe brain injury or dementia. Its effects may be acute, chronic, or transient. The delusions center around one of the senses—most often sight—and remain localized to that one sense. For example, a man afflicted with Capgras may recognize his wife's voice on the phone yet believe that she is an impostor when he sees her in person.

Whatever the cause in Frances's case, she no longer recognized her son. She confused him with his father (her husband), who had passed away six years earlier. She could no longer process the recollection of her son the way she had before dementia damaged her short-term memories. The son had tried to bring his mom into his reality by explaining that he was her son, but his mother met his efforts with anger and anxiety. He told me that his mother would respond more positively and be more cooperative if he just "went along with her perception and did not argue with her about his identity." He had come to realize through trial and error that he could not win this dispute. Letting go of the need to try to convince his mother of his identity had paradoxically given him a greater feeling of empowerment.

We all forget things occasionally, but the short-term memory loss caused by dementia is different. The following paragraphs describe how our brains usually store short-term and long-term memories, and how dementia affects our normal memory storage processes.

Imagine a short-term memory file cabinet appearing every morning on the outer edge of your brain for the memories you will create today—what you ate for breakfast, where you parked your car when you arrived at work, and so on. At the end of the day, this cabinet will move in one notch, toward the center of your brain, and be replaced by a new outer-edge file cabinet the next day (and the next, and the next). These more recent files contain the short-term memories. Each file cabinet, as it ages, moves deeper and deeper into the recesses of the brain. As these cabinets age, they become the long-term memories.

The ongoing destruction caused by the dementia begins to destroy these files, however, starting with today's file cabinet.

How does it feel to have these recent memories destroyed? Consider this comparison: almost all of us have gone to the mall, parked, shopped, and returned to the lot only to realize we cannot remember where we left the car. You know how uncomfortable it feels when you can't find your car? You may even start to wonder if it has been stolen. Well, that unpleasant blank feeling and memory deficit is what the dementia-challenged adult feels every day, every hour, every minute. Can you imagine how frightening and disorienting this must be?

If we continue to visualize the rows of memory storage files in the "memory room" of our brains, with the most recent memories in front and the long-ago memories farther and farther back, we can begin to understand how dementia-challenged people lose the ability to access the most recent memories. The fluid (short-term) memory file cabinets disappear, one by one.

Yet people with dementia often maintain the ability to access memories from long ago (known as "crystal memories"), because many of those far-back memory storage files have not yet been deleted by the dementia. Many family caregivers have told me that their family members with dementia can clearly remember detailed events from long ago but cannot remember things that happened yesterday. This is a common experience. It is as if people with dementia are on "rewind" in their memories, like a biographical movie running backwards. Short-term memories start to disappear, while long-ago memories become clearer and may feel like "now," making it easier to confuse twenty-year-old or thirty-year-old memories with the present time.

Understanding how memories are stored and lost makes it easier to understand the memory loss of dementia and how it affects people with dementia every day. Their world becomes a puzzling mix-up of times, feelings, and visions from their past life randomly woven into the present. The good news is that you can still share meaningful moments with your loved one.

Often, we initially think about the dementia only as memory loss. Yet, it is so much more complex than just memory loss, as the functions needed to "think" about memory—to understand and process the information that actually makes it a memory—are quite complex. When you retrieve a memory from the part of your brain where it is stored, your brain also goes to work to recapture, arrange, and process the bits and pieces of information that make the "memory storyline" make sense, such as:

- Where it happened?
- When it happened?
- Why it happened?
- Who was with you?
- How did it make you feel at that time? (Sad, happy, scared, alone, safe, etc.)
- What did you see?
- What did you hear?
- What did you touch?

When you retrieve these bits and pieces of the storyline your brain instantly advances into thinking mode, sorting out each detail and discerning how all of this made you feel then and how it makes you feel now as you remember. This automatic cognitive response and intellectual interpretation would play out differently if you had gaps in this information, if this entire step-by-step process of thinking started to unravel. What if your detailed vision of what happened was no longer clear? You would not be able to think of who was there with you. Some or all of the sounds might now be muffled, partial, or nonexistent. How would you manage all of this information if the thinking/reasoning/processing procedures you have followed effortlessly before the loss of brain function are now all distorted, muddled, or even hijacked by a cause of dementia? Would this make you feel different? You might begin to feel as if it never really happened or begin to confabulate the details to help the jumbled elements of the memory make sense. Your unconscious mind would attempt to fill in the gaps, perhaps swapping in an old memory or detail in order to come up with a conceivable alternative.

When people hear the word "dementia" they often think of dementia only as memory loss. Although there is the probability of having memory loss, I want you to understand there is much more to the dementia journey than just losing a memory. Even if a memory, or parts of it remain, if you are unable to understand or process it, you won't be able to make use of it. It becomes empty and useless information. And, as a matter of fact, with some causes of dementia symptoms, memory is not affected at all.

As you read the information below, you will better understand that, although memory loss does constitute painful and recognizable decline, there are many dementia symptoms that are often more perplexing, heartrending, and misunderstood than just the loss of a memory.

The following information from the Alzheimer's Association provides additional details about dementia symptoms.

Information Compiled by Denise Davis, Program Director, Alzheimer's Association's Greater Sacramento Area Office.

Memory loss that disrupts everyday life is not a normal part of aging. However, there is no clear line that separates normal changes from the warning signs. Because of this uncertainty about what's causing a problem, if a loved one's abilities seem to be declining, it is a good idea to get a diagnosis from a doctor—and from a doctor who specializes in diagnosing dementia, if possible.

According to the Alzheimer's Association, these are the ten warning signs of dementia:

1. *Memory Loss.* This is when a person's immediate memory is being challenged. Forgetting recently learned information is one of the most common signs of dementia.
2. *Difficulty Performing Familiar Tasks.* People with dementia often find it hard to plan or complete everyday tasks. Individuals may lose track of the steps involved in preparing a meal, placing a telephone call, or playing a game.
3. *Problems with Language.* People with Alzheimer disease may often forget simple words or substitute unusual

words, making their speech or writing hard to understand. They may be unable to find the fork, for example, and instead ask for "that thing for my mouth."

4. *Disorientation to Time and Place.* Persons with Alzheimer disease can become lost in their own neighborhoods, forget where they are and how they got there, and not know how to get back home.

5. *Poor or Decreased Judgment.* Those with Alzheimer's may dress inappropriately, wearing several layers on a warm day or little clothing in the cold. They may show poor judgment about money, like giving away large sums to telemarketers.

6. *Problems with Abstract Thinking.* Someone with Alzheimer disease may have unusual difficulty performing complex mental tasks; for example, they may forget what numbers are and how they should be used.

7. *Misplacing Things.* A person with Alzheimer disease may put things in unusual places—a high-heeled shoe in the freezer or a necklace in the sugar bowl.

8. *Changes in Mood or Behavior.* Someone with Alzheimer disease may show rapid mood swings—from calm to tears to anger—for no apparent reason.

9. *Changes in Personality.* The personalities of people with dementia can change dramatically. They may become extremely confused, suspicious, fearful, or dependent on a family member.

10. *Loss of Initiative.* A person with Alzheimer disease may become very passive, sitting in front of the TV for hours, sleeping more than usual, or not wanting to do normal activities.

Dementia is a general term for a group of brain disorders, and Alzheimer's is the most common type of dementia, accounting for 60 to 80 percent of those with dementia.

How can you tell whether someone's symptoms are a sign of normal aging or are a sign of dementia? There are some specific signs. For example, all types of dementia involve mental decline that

- is a step down from a higher level of functioning (for example, the person did not always have a poor memory);
- is severe enough to interfere with usual activities and daily life; and
- affects more than one of the following four core mental abilities:
  - recent memory (the ability to learn and recall new information)
  - language (the ability to write or speak, or to understand written or spoken words)
  - visuospatial function (the brain's ability to translate visual signals into an accurate impression of where objects are located in space, and the ability to understand and use symbols, maps, etc.)
  - executive function (the ability to plan, reason, solve problems, and focus on a task).

There are over one hundred types of dementia. Some of the more widely known types are

- Alzheimer disease
- mild cognitive impairment (MCI), a pre-dementia state
- mixed dementia: Alzheimer disease and vascular dementia occurring at the same time
- dementia with Lewy body (Lewy body dementia)
- Parkinson's disease
- frontotemporal dementia (Pick's disease)
- Creutzfeldt-Jakob disease (CJD)
- normal pressure hydrocephalus (NPH)
- Huntington's disease (HD)
- Wernicke-Korsakoff syndrome

The various types of dementia have different warning signs, rates of progression, and behaviors, which is one reason it's important to get an accurate diagnosis of the type of dementia. An accurate diagnosis means that the person with dementia and his or her caregivers can learn more about the likely (though not certain) progression in a person with that specific kind of dementia. Medications can help relieve some of the more troubling behaviors for certain kinds of dementia; these medications are especially useful when behavior modification techniques (such as those described in this book) are not effective enough.

Progressive types of dementia, including Alzheimer disease, affect key thought processes, including the following six areas:

1. *Memory.* A person with a failing memory may not, for example, be able to keep in mind that getting dressed and getting into a car is a sequence leading up to dinner with friends. Events begin to exist on their own, without being linked to other events. None has a larger context.

2. *Language/communication.* The ability to communicate is what allows us to connect with others in the world, to get and give information of all sorts. We rely on communication to express needs and feelings. Language is the most obvious form of communication, but there are other ways of communicating too. We rely on gestures, body language, and facial expressions. Through dementia, the ability to communicate is gradually lost. The first problem is usually with word finding; people struggle to find the right word for the situation, such as the appropriate word in a conversation. They may forget names of people who are well-known to them. Later, they may have difficulty expressing ideas; they may know what they want to say but not be able to find the words. All of this can lead to embarrassment and frustration, possibly prompting the person to withdraw. Communication difficulties and frustrations can produce emotional outbursts. Some people with the problem blame caregivers.

3. *Reasoning.* People with dementia cannot be reasonable. Most of us expect others to be reasonable, and we assume that they will be reasonable when we interact with them. Throughout daily life, we regularly appeal to reason, and we employ logic and persuasion in many situations. And we expect others to use logic and persuasion

in return. Most of all, we expect that these forms of interaction will carry the day. Dementia turns these expectations upside down. Increasingly, normal forms of interaction—like persuasion—will not work. Logic will fail and may backfire. Asking the person to think ahead through a series of steps may cause confusion, withdrawal, or impetuous behavior. As the person with dementia loses his or her reasoning power, the caregiver will need to take more control.

4. *Judgment.* Judgment is the ability we use when we ask the question, "What if?" Asking ourselves this question allows us to judge the safety, benefits, and drawbacks of a situation. The ability to imagine the possible outcomes of a situation is very important for personal safety. Unfortunately, this capacity is lost relatively early in dementia. Because of distorted thinking, judgment may be poor or faulty and utterly different from the person's previous decision-making abilities and behaviors. The person's own insight into his or her thinking problems varies greatly among individuals, and changes as the disease advances. At first, the person with dementia may be cognizant that he or she has a problem; later, he or she will not realize that there is a problem. All of this makes it hard to know whether and how much to involve the person in critical life choices.

5. *Abstract thought.* We rely on abstract thought to deal with everything in our lives that is not concrete. In fact, numerous things we take for granted are abstract. Numbers and directions are abstract, as is time. The past and the future are held in order by the power of abstraction. Possibilities are abstract, including the ability to think about the "what ifs" in our lives. Being able to know "where" and "how much" is part of abstraction, and so are relationships—the connections we share among family members and friends. Like the other powers of thought, abstraction declines with the progression of dementia. Again, this ability is lost fairly early in the disease, which means that many of the concepts we rely on to live in this world no longer have meaning for the person who has dementia.

6. *Perception.* Normal perception involves two features. First, our senses allow us to take in the world around us. Through sight and hearing, and also through touch, smell, and taste, we take note of things outside of ourselves. Second, our brains make sense out of what we

observe. People with dementia often make mistakes in sensing and interpreting things. For example, they may interpret images on television as being real and start talking back to them. Reflections, including a person's own reflection in a mirror, can be mistaken for real people who suddenly appear and disappear. Patterns in floor tile or carpets can be mistaken for holes that need to be stepped over or avoided. They may even be seen as uncrossable barriers. Such misperceptions are sometimes called pseudo-hallucinations. Since the root causes of pseudo-hallucinations may actually be situated in poor hearing or eyesight, testing and correcting hearing and visual problems can sometimes help. However, even when the person who has dementia is able to see and hear clearly, he or she may still be unable to interpret things accurately.

Frances continued on her dementia journey with her son by her side for three more years. Her activity level declined slowly over that time, and her son needed more and more help from professional care providers. Frances's physical care needs escalated, and he wasn't able to provide for all of her needs on his own.

I continue to admire the countless family care providers who step up to dedicate months and even years to caring for parents, siblings, spouses, or even nonrelatives, making sure that the person with dementia is led along a path strewn with feelings of safety, security, love, and with shared meaningful moments. Frances's son confided in me at her memorial service that although this had been the most difficult time in his adult life, it had cemented a unique bond in his relationship with his mother. He was experiencing mixed emotions: sadness at her loss, comfort that she was no longer suffering, and a strange feeling of "what do I do now?" because he had also lost his role as a full-time caregiver. Many care providers face this same roller coaster of emotions at the end of the dementia care journey, which is another reason that it's important to ask for assistance all along the way.

CHAPTER SIX

Jill

Into the Dementia Wonderland

One day at an art gallery, Jill was studying a beautiful painting of a beach, with shimmering sand, deep aqua waves, and an airy cottage with two empty beach chairs facing the dazzling blue ocean. As she stood there looking at the artist's work, she began to cry. The gallery owner came up and introduced herself, asking if she could be of assistance.

Jill replied, "My name is Jill, and my mother has advanced dementia. I am her full-time caregiver, and she seems to be getting further and further away from me as her disease progresses. The 'place' where she seems to go most often in her mind is a beach cottage she often mentioned when reminiscing about her childhood. That place seems to be very much like the place in this painting. I want to buy it and hang it in my mother's room so she and I can 'visit' this special place from her long-ago memories."

The art gallery owner was so touched by Jill's deep connection with her mother that she helped her purchase the painting on a payment plan. This simple act beautifully enriched the time Jill shared with her mother.

Lessons Learned

You will never win an argument with someone who has dementia. In fact, you may already sense that the person you are caring for will be much more cooperative if you acknowledge and give *affirmative responses* to his or her feelings and subsequent behaviors—in *his or her reality*, not in yours. This reality, from which the person who has dementia may drift in and out, is very different from your reality and from what your loved one's reality was before the dementia became an issue.

Here are two examples of affirmative responses to challenging behaviors:

1. Mr. Jones has been living in a secured memory care environment for several weeks. He keeps trying to leave through the secure door. He becomes very agitated if the care staff tells him that he cannot go out that door. He even gets aggressive with caregivers who say, "No, you can't go out this door." Care staff found the solution by redirecting him with affirming statements such as, "I am so sorry, but this door is out of order. The door in back is operating. Let me show you the way." The back door led out to the secure courtyard, and Mr. Jones could go in and out as he pleased.

2. When an adult with dementia and memory loss is asking for a loved one whom you know passed away several years ago, you are in a difficult situation. Instead of trying to bring the person into the painful reality of the loss of the loved one and causing him to experience unresolved temporary grieving, you can "reminisce" with him about the person who is no longer with him. You might ask: "When was the last time you saw her?" "How long has it been since you talked with him?" "What was your favorite time you spent together?" "Where did you first meet?"

   As you become more and more dementia-aware you may recognize that the adult with dementia who you are "reminiscing" with has passed the point of being able to effortlessly process questions and will feel less anxious if you use a simpler "feeling prompt" approach. Instead of asking, "When was the last time you saw her?" Try a positive feeling trigger statement such as, "You enjoyed spending time with her" or "It feels good to think about time with her." Making a statement rather than asking a question helps to "cue the person" to the feeling in the moment. It reduces the need for him to struggle with the fragmented thinking about how he might have felt or should have felt. Spend a few meaningful moments with the person affirming past memories and feelings. Most of the time he will go on to other thoughts, and neither of you will have to experience the loss and grief over and over again.

I like to relate the "reality" of the person with dementia to the notion of "reality" in the book *Alice in Wonderland.* If you are familiar with the story, you know that Alice stepped through the looking-glass mirror to another world, a fantasy "reality" she called a "wonder-land," where she enjoyed amazing adventures with the Cheshire Cat, the White Rabbit, and many other interesting characters. When she stepped back through the mirror into the reality of the parlor in her home, however, she could not bring her new friends or unusual adventures with her. They did not exist in this world.

The most challenging behaviors for caregivers sometimes are precipitated by their attempts to bring the person who has dementia into their own reality. These attempts can stir up anxiety, anger, fear, combativeness, and aggression in the person receiving care. As caregivers, we can more easily connect if we confidently step through that person's "mirror" into her world and allow her to act as our "Alice"— to lead us through the dementia wonderland.

Remember: the feelings remain long after the event has been forgotten! I love the way Maya Angelou expressed this: "I've learned that people will forget what you said, people will forget what you did, but people will never forget how you made them feel."

You have probably experienced a variety of behaviors—some pleasant and some not so pleasant—from the person in your care. Although you may not be able to identify or understand the cause of the behavior at the time, you might keep in mind that there is a reason for every behavior. As the person who has dementia travels back into his past, he experiences the emotions attached to long-ago memories just as if these past events were occurring in the present. How he acts reflects how he felt *then*. In other words, long-ago emotions are influencing current actions.

If these feelings are based on memories that cause fear, anger, or insecurity, the person who has dementia will "act out" negative behaviors—for example, by resisting your requests. Your loved one or client may say or do unkind or hurtful things, or she may cry and attempt to burden you with guilt or grief. On the other hand, if the feelings are rooted in memories of joy, happiness, and security, she will tend to be kinder and more cooperative.

Additionally, the more at peace you are, the more easily you will guide your loved one or client into a place of serenity. In the next chapter, we explore further how important it is for the caregiver to be in a "happy place." The caregiver who remains calm can gently lead the person who has dementia to experience feelings of peace.

Perceptions and Approaches

Even the most challenging and bizarre dementia behaviors are born from past events. These behaviors are triggered by things that are happening now that in some way evoke a sight, smell, sound, or emotion from long ago. When you understand the root causes of these behaviors, you can put on your creative thinking cap and develop unique approaches that will help you redirect your loved one or client into more cooperative behaviors.

Even if you do not know what's causing a specific behavior, you can still use redirection to obtain a more tranquil reaction, as long as you approach each challenge from a place of peacefulness.

Family caregivers usually have no choice but to take on the challenges of caregiving. Life is suddenly interrupted. Caregivers respond in a variety of ways, but very few caregivers find that taking care of someone with dementia is undemanding, as comments like these remind us:

- "I took care of my mom for three years. It was the most difficult time in my life."
- "I took care of my wife for two years. We had to place her in a memory care facility for the last year. That was the hardest thing I've ever had to do."
- "My husband and I had so many plans for our retirement years. We were about four years away and had just started building our retirement home when he was diagnosed with Alzheimer's. We finished our home early, but we had to forget all the other plans we had. After he died, I had to sell the house— there were just too many things to remind me of those difficult years."

Remaining calm while caring for the person who has dementia can be very difficult. The stress that caregivers face is considered chronic stress because it is long-term, constant, and unrelenting. This stress can be powerful enough to damage the caregiver's health and cause serious illness. Properly managing stress is vital to successful caregiving.

This chapter's message is simple: one way to manage stress is to remember that you cannot correct the dementia wonderland. All attempts to bring people with dementia into "reality" will only create more stress for both parties. Instead of setting yourself up for intense frustration, give your loved one or client *affirmative responses and positive action statements*. Doing so will help you remain in a place of calm confidence, which will in turn help the person who has dementia.

CHAPTER SEVEN

Natalie

Much More than Words

Natalie and George had been married fifty-seven years and had raised two sons and a daughter. When George was diagnosed with dementia and suffered a rapid cognitive decline, the family banded together to try to keep him at home. The sons and daughter were busy with their families and jobs, so most of the caregiving fell on Natalie's shoulders.

As the dementia began manifesting itself in more challenging ways, Natalie began to fail both physically and mentally. And then the level of care that George needed increased significantly, way beyond what anyone in the family could provide. George had traveled so far back into his past memories that he could not remember his children or Natalie; he began to yell at them to get out of the house. He saw his family as strangers and felt threatened by them. Finally, he grew so anxious and paranoid that the family knew it was time to place him in a secured environment that could provide the kind of care he now needed.

Natalie faithfully visited George in his new home. Her visits were appreciated by both George and the staff, but George continued to revert back to a time in his past where he could not remember who she was. He would sit and hold her hand during the visits, sharing what he could of his memories as they smiled and chatted. But he would only call Natalie "the nice lady." The children also visited and were welcomed in the same way, as nice strangers.

Early one morning, George made his way to the nurse's station and leaned over the counter to speak to the night nurse on duty. With tears in his eyes he told her, "Natalie came and kissed me goodbye last night." The nurse was startled, "You remember Natalie?" George smiled and shuffled back to his room. The look on his face appeared to signal that he had just shared a special secret.

Just hours earlier, Natalie had been killed in an automobile accident. At the time George spoke to the nurse, though, neither the nurse nor anyone in the memory care facility had been informed of the heart-breaking news. How did George know? Did Natalie kiss him goodnight? We will never know what clued George into sensing this tragedy.

Natalie and George's story was shared with me by one of their sons. When he finished, we wept together with tears rolling down our cheeks. It was clear how truly powerful the human heart-to-heart connection is.

Lessons Learned

When connecting to their intense past feelings and memories, people with dementia tap into a deeper level of communication. In fact, they communicate in ways that we, as caregivers, often cannot see or understand by normal means. People with dementia may attempt to compensate for the loss of traditional ways of communicating—such as speech—in order to understand the confusing world around them.

According to Albert Mehrabian, professor emeritus of psychology at the University of California, Los Angeles, communication with the person who has dementia is only 7 percent verbal. The other 93 percent of communication is conveyed through our tone of voice, our body language, our approach (physically moving into that person's "space" to interact), and our emotions. These signals are all "heard" and interpreted loudly and clearly by people with cognitive impairment.

As the disease strips away their language centers, people with dementia lose their ability to communicate verbally. The brain attempts to compensate for these losses by using all of the remaining senses to perceive, interpret, and acknowledge what is happening in each person's immediate surroundings. The use of other senses heightens the impact of nonverbal communication.

In summary, the person who has dementia will feel what you are feeling and reflect those emotions back.

During a training session for staff at a memory care facility, one of the residents wheeled herself into the dining room where we were conducting the training. She stopped her wheelchair right next to me. One of the staff got up and wanted to take her back into the hall, but I asked the staff member to return to her seat. I reached for the resident's hand.

The resident took my hand and looked up at me. I asked her if she wanted to join us. She smiled and said, "Yes, it feels warm next to you!" I asked her if she knew what I was feeling, and she said, "I think so. I think you are feeling happy, and I am too!"

Just before the resident came in, I had been sharing information about the importance of being in your "happy place" as a caregiver. Since the person who has dementia mirrors our emotions, if we are happy and have a pleasant demeanor, we will help the person with dementia be in their "happy place" as often as possible. This resident could feel my calm, just as she would soon begin to sense the positive emotions in all the staff who had attended the session and quickly began applying this technique.

The best way to help the person who has dementia remain calm is for you to remain calm. Do your best to leave harassed or anxious feelings outside of the relationship. Above all, take time away to find respite and keep yourself in a less stressed place. Even if you are not filled with happiness, you can still smile and make eye contact. Setting the right tone at the beginning of every interaction will result in a higher level of cooperation from the person who has dementia.

In sharp contrast to the above example, I once conducted an in-home assessment for a couple in which the wife had a dementia diagnosis. I arrived at the porch and was about to knock when I heard quite a scuffle inside. The wife was screaming at the top of her lungs, "Get out, get out, get out of my house, you b——! Leave me alone!"

I knocked loudly, and the husband answered the door looking very embarrassed. He anxiously let me in, saying, "Please excuse my wife. She is having a very bad day and does not want the visiting nurse to take her vitals. Can you help her, Laura?"

I came around the corner to find the visiting nurse in a distressed state. She was trying hopelessly to grab the uncooperative patient's arm: "Now, you have to calm down. I need to take your blood pressure, and I am late for my next appointment. You should not be calling me names. Let me get this done now. Calm down this instant!"

The wife was having no part of the nurse's pushiness and arrogance. Instead, the ninety-four-pound wife swung her tiny arms and kicked at the nurse while screaming foul words at the top of her lungs. I calmly asked the nurse if she could come back after her next appointment, explaining that I would work on calming her patient before she returned. The nurse was indignant: "She might try to hit or kick you, so watch out!" I assured her I would be okay.

As the nurse left the room, I took a deep breath, quickly surveyed the situation, and discerned that the nurse's frantic, pushy approach was a big factor in the wife's combativeness and resistance. Even in her dementia confusion, the wife sensed the nurse's frustration, which was making the wife feel apprehensive about this unfamiliar person in her house. Consider: here was a complete stranger who had come into her personal space and had been grabbing her and scolding her.

I recognized that I could help to make this agitated wife feel calmer and safe and secure only if I approached her slowly and serenely, overemphasizing a sense of tranquility as I came within reach of her and presenting a hushed, relaxed, composed, and gentle demeanor. I sat down next to the enraged woman and softly spoke as she kept up her frantic gestures and angry words: "I will go away as you ask, but I am so tired. I know that you do not want me here, but may I sit next to you and rest for just a minute? I have come a long way and need to sit in your lovely home and rest. I am soooo tired."

I spoke these words several times as slowly and as softly as I could, just loud enough so she could hear me. My words grew even softer, and she hesitated and listened. Her words also softened, and she started to relax. I took a deep breath and went quiet. Then she became quiet, and within a few minutes she fell sound asleep next to me.

When there are changes in the brain that affect memory, reasoning, and language, the primary tool of communication for the person who has dementia becomes behavior. Dementia may completely change a person's mood and personality. At first, memory loss and difficulty in thinking clearly may bother the person who has dementia. Later, disruptive behavior and other problems may start, and the person may not even be aware of what he or she is doing.

Caregiving is stressful, both emotionally and physically. Not only do many caregivers feed, bathe, and provide emotional support, but they do most of the daily household maintenance as well. According to the Family Caregiver Alliance, 22 percent of caregivers report feeling exhausted at night. Unfortunately, the more stressed you are, the more stressed the person who has dementia is likely to become. The good news is that serenity can draw out wonderfully pleasant behavior.

Perceptions and Approaches

The person with dementia is hypersensitive to what you are feeling. For example, a 2009 study by C. M. Kipps and others showed that people with dementia can no longer distinguish between verbal sarcasm and truth. Instead, they rely heavily on the feelings that come with the words. When faced with sarcasm, they will ignore any verbal misrepresentation from the speaker and will instead "read" the truth of the other person's feelings. If you sarcastically tell someone with dementia, "Oh, don't worry—I'm feeling just *fine*," he or she will probably see right through it.

My experiences have proven this over and over. The person who has dementia will understand how we feel better than they will understand what we say. If you are angry or anxious, how is the person you are caring for likely to feel? If you are frustrated and intolerant, what type of behavior will you get back from him or her? And if you are tired and burned out, how can you expect the person you are caring for to feel cooperative and helpful?

It is not only important that you care for yourself for your own sake; it is equally important to care for yourself so that you can help your loved one or client cope with this devastating disease. Since the person with dementia will mirror your feelings and moods, you have the power to set the tone. Assuming an upbeat manner will create many more positive moments for you both as you go about your day. If you can do it, you will be rewarded with an enhanced caregiving relationship.

CHAPTER EIGHT

Vada

Past, Present, and Future

One of the requirements for my gerontology degree was a delightful course called "Reminiscence." Every student was paired with a skilled nursing facility resident who had been diagnosed with some form of dementia. This person was to be our "partner" for the semester.

We would meet for class at the facility and spend the first hour with our partners, getting to know them and establishing rapport and a trusting relationship. They had varying degrees of dementia, but most seemed to enjoy the attention and time that we gave them. After the first hour, we would lead our residents down to a common area—the activity room—and we would all sit in a circle to participate in the group portion of class, called "reminiscence."

Each day we would have a planned theme, or topic, to spark memories and story sharing as a group. Almost everyone enjoyed the discussions of such topics as "your wedding day," "the war years," and "childhood pets."

One resident, however, did not seem to appreciate the opportunity to share. She was not showing much enthusiasm for our visits or activities. The resident's name was Vada, and her reputation preceded her.

From the beginning, the student paired with Vada had known she was in for a challenge. Vada was 101 years old and in very poor health with a terminal illness. She spoke to the staff in an abrasive way and was constantly complaining about the facility, the food, the care, and nearly every person within a 10-foot radius.

Vada was angry and anxious, and she resisted all attempts to make her last days comfortable and happy. Hard of hearing, she had loud outbursts during the group memory activity: "What are we doing here?" "I can't hear them. What did they say?" "Take me back to my room!"

This behavior went on time after time until the day our topic was "birthdays." As we went around the circle asking how people had celebrated their childhood birthdays or what their favorite birthday was, we came to Vada. To our shock, we were not greeted by the usual angry protest. In a quiet, shaky voice full of emotion, she began telling us about her eighth birthday.

She grew up poor as an only child on an isolated farm on the midwestern plains. Her father and mother worked hard from sunup to sundown, and Vada was also expected to contribute by doing loads of chores. She did not attend school. Her mother did her best to homeschool her in reading, writing, and arithmetic.

Because there were no other children nearby, Vada had few chances to play or socialize with anyone her own age. One morning, about six months before Vada's eighth birthday, her mother surprised her with the news that they could throw a big birthday bash for her! Over the next six months, Vada and her mother created handwritten invitations that her father took to children throughout the county. Together they baked, made homemade decorations, and spent many days in anticipation of the big celebration.

As Vada described the preparations, her face lit up, and she related what she remembered. All of the participants in the class were mesmerized at the uncharacteristic change in her behavior, and we wanted to hear more. Suddenly, Vada began to cry, and her voice got even softer. On the day of her birthday, she jumped out of bed and ran to the window of the farmhouse. She was greeted with the sight of blinding, drifting snow. Because of the blizzard, no one could come to the party.

The pain and disappointment from years before were written on Vada's face, and the tears rolled freely. She looked around the room, "I hate being alone. My family is gone. I am sick and lonely. Please don't let me die here all alone." That was the first time as a student that I had experienced the phenomenon of a person who has dementia reliving past memories and feelings. We all rallied and did our best to comfort Vada.

At our next class, we brought her a very large stuffed bear that we had all autographed with comforting phrases: "We love you, Vada." "We are here for you." "You are not alone." She took that bear into her arms and beamed.

The following week, the staff came to our class and informed us that Vada had passed away with a contented smile, still holding her soft, furry friend in her arms.

Lessons Learned

As the short-term memory fades, a person with dementia sometimes becomes caught up in painful, unresolved memories and is trapped by the negative feelings those memories trigger. This "rut" may be the root behind unpleasant behaviors.

Many people who have dementia appreciate it when someone does something as simple as listening with a caring ear. They may express painful feelings that they are still trying to work through. When you adjust your listening skills to accommodate both the pleasant and the painful memories—listening without judgment or argument—you will become much more effective at communicating and speaking the special "dialect of dementia." This kind of listening can also create an opening for the person with dementia to resolve or tie up loose ends by working through the negative events, venting "emotional steam" that may have been suppressed for years. It sometimes even happens that the person will go back in time to escape the painful *present* reality, only to get stuck in equally painful long-ago memories.

But as we experienced with Vada, being able to share lonely and frightened feelings with other people who show true concern and empathy can help a person release those feelings and experience a more meaningful and secure life passage.

Perceptions and Approaches

When you are communicating with someone with dementia, be patient and develop a trusting relationship. Always provide a dignified and respectful atmosphere, even if the person is not always able to provide the same for you.

Each dementia journey is characterized and navigated by the person's unique personality and history, so we must provide our loved ones and clients with direction. This direction must be based upon a deeper understanding of *their distinctive courses.* Although those with dementia have much in common in terms of the disease of dementia, each individual brings a one-of-a-kind storyline, so it is up to the caregiver to listen, adjust, and change, remaining flexible and fluid in addressing the ever-evolving needs as the dementia progresses.

Sometimes the stories that the person with dementia shares will be unclear, repetitive, or even dull. However, the more time you take to show genuine interest—intently focusing on what the person can share with you about his or her past—the better able you will be to build a deep connection. This connection will, in turn, help you develop care solutions that effectively meet the social and emotional needs of your client or loved one.

Vada is a prime example. Because our class was able to hear her story and heal her wounded heart, we were able to give her the compassion she needed before her passing.

Human beings, including human beings with dementia, need to be able to express their feelings to someone who cares; this is especially true of strong (and perhaps unpleasant) feelings from one's past. The strong feelings that are directly connected to past memories do not magically evaporate as we age. On the contrary, they often come back late in life to haunt us, just as we observed when Vada relived the agonizing sentiments associated with her eighth birthday. By listening for and catching an emotion that may have been bottled up inside someone for years, we allow the person to express those feelings and ease their minds and hearts.

CHAPTER NINE

Joe

Communicating the Gift of Value

Recently I was asked to consult at a local skilled nursing facility to assist with a new resident who was being very uncooperative. He would not allow the staff to guide him to the dining area for meals or to his room for sleep, and he was exhibiting a puzzling, repetitive behavior. I will call this dear fellow Joe.

When I arrived, the staff led me to a long hallway where I saw Joe shuffling along and feeling the hallway walls, reaching as high as he could and as low as he could, muttering to himself as he studied the spot of wall in front of him. Up and down the long hall, back and forth he went. When the staff would come alongside and ask him to come for lunch, he would give them an emphatic "No!" and go back to his task with complete focus.

He made no attempt to converse with the staff, and there were no family or friends we could talk with to find out what might be causing his unusual actions, so I asked to see his chart. The chart gave me an idea of where he was in his past reality.

Utilizing a tool called *reflective action*, I stood very near to him and began to "mirror his actions" as we moved together on the wall. I moved at his pace and did exactly what he did. Then after a few moments, I stopped and touched the back of his hand, moving directly in front of him and taking both of his hands in mine. I looked into his eyes and asked him, "Joe, do you see this? Someone has done a very poor job on the finish of this wall. We need to get our best repairman here to refinish it. Who would be the best man for this job?" He looked intently into my eyes and answered, "Frank!"

I quickly asked him, "Where is Frank?" He still had his hands in mine as we both turned our heads this way and that, visually searching for Frank. When it was clear that Frank was not immediately at hand, I looked at my watch and said, "Oh, it's lunchtime. Frank has taken his usual lunch break. Let's go get our lunch, and we can get Frank to fix this wall first thing this afternoon."

Joe took my outstretched arm and shuffled down to the dining area. I sat with him while he ate lunch and told me about his work.

The staff asked, "Laura, how did you get him to do that?"

I replied, "I simply visited Joe in his past memories of his occupation, as a creative and artistic wall finisher! He was a specialist as an Italian wall finisher, a craft he learned from his father and brought over to our country when his family immigrated here. He is beautifying and fixing your walls for you!" And as soon as he was done eating lunch, off he went, back to "work," visiting a place that gave him feelings of pride and self-worth.

A few weeks later, I called to follow up and was pleased to hear that this technique worked well for ongoing cooperation whenever the staff felt it was needed. The staff had even gone a creative step further! One evening as it was getting late and a staff member was attempting to get Joe to his room for bed, she encountered some resistance. She told Joe that if they requested help from Frank at this late hour, they would probably have to pay him overtime. Joe's eyes widened, "Oh, no! No overtime!" He immediately followed her to his room for the night.

And Joe gave another *affirmative response* when the staff implemented a successful plan every day at lunchtime. A staff member simply brought him his lunch in an old-fashioned metal lunchbox. He would carry it to the dining room and oblige the staff by calmly consuming his meal with little or no resistance. The old lunchbox triggered images of his past noontime routine, giving him the sense of security and familiarity he was searching for.

Lessons Learned

If you were confused about your surroundings, could not remember who the people near you were, felt disoriented and overwhelmed, and could only access memories and feelings from your distant past, where would you go to feel the most secure and content? Of course, back in time, to memories that brought you happiness, delight, and feelings of self-worth and purpose.

In contrast, if you had frightening or unhappy feelings driven by painful memories, you would naturally want to avoid those unpleasant stops on your journey. However, as we saw with Vada in the last chapter, the person who has dementia may become "stuck" in those negative unresolved memories and feelings. Understanding the person's behavior helps reveal whether he or she is experiencing pleasant or unpleasant memories. If someone is experiencing negative feelings, we want to affirm the person and yet bring comfort and peace to the situation. Conversely, when the person is in a good place, we want to help reinforce the positive memories and feelings.

Remember: you will never win an argument with a person who has dementia. But whenever you affirm the emotions that the person is experiencing, you will instead enjoy a magical connection! Affirming emotions will provide many wonderful opportunities for you both to feel appreciated. Joe's story illustrates how we all respond in an affirmative way when we are directed toward positive feelings. Making people with dementia feel valued helps create an emotional safe place for them to land amidst their confusion.

The brain and the memory storage processes are extraordinarily complex. They are made up of several distinct parts, and every part has its own function. While there are many different storage portions of the brain, they all have different functions, and all of the parts of the brain must work together to complete even the simplest task. As dementia affects each area of the brain, certain functions or abilities can be lost, and the brain will then attempt to compensate for the loss, desperately trying to make sense of the ongoing confusion. When one or more dots in the connect-the-dots schematic are missing, the person is in need of help or a coping mechanism to complete even a common or familiar task.

Further, changes in behavior and changes in the person's inability to communicate may be related to damage caused by the disease. He or she may experience many bewildering feelings but not have the ability to express them verbally.

Perceptions and Approaches

Our usual ways of communicating become less effective as the dementia progresses. Communicating effectively with a person who has dementia requires skill, confidence, and adaptability. Approach each situation with patience. Repeat phrases that produce an *affirmative response*. Slow down, watch, and listen—and repeat, repeat, repeat. Use creativity to express both your feelings and your message. Practice these new skills to convey your message effectively and to feel confident when you handle each difficult situation.

Look back on how we connected with Joe. Through *reflective action*, we mirrored his physical actions and showed him that we were on his side and working to enter his world rather than bring him into ours. After that, the door was open to communicate with him verbally.

When you want to communicate with your loved one or client, be sure to get the person's attention and make eye contact. Make certain the person feels that he or she is your only focus. Look him or her directly in the eye and be totally present. Speak slowly and clearly, giving only one message at a time. Limit outside distractions such as a TV or radio.

Use actions as well as words—the old "show and tell" skills that you learned as a child in school. For example, if you are going out for a walk with your loved one or client, hand the person a sweater and point at the door at the same time, saying that it is time for his or her walk.

Even when their communication abilities are failing, you can still show people that you understand their unique attempts to get across what they wish to share. Watch facial and bodily responses. The person's reaction to what you say can give you an idea of how much he or she understands. Respond to his or her moods and emotions, especially when the words do not make sense or are inappropriate.

And finally, never lose sight of the importance of nonverbal cues. We all communicate by emotion, expression, and touch. Holding a hand, or smiling when talking, can convey much more than any words.

We all want to be heard, validated, and valued. The following story beautifully illustrates how important it is to bring value to the person who has dementia.

Lessons from Hazel
By Deana Chitambar, RN, CHPN

The many facets of my job as a hospice registered nurse include teaching a class on Alzheimer disease at dementia care facilities. My students are professional caregivers who are responsible for assisting residents with activities of daily living (ADLs), such as dressing, toileting, and bathing.

One day in class, we were having an interesting discussion on the definition and diagnosis of Alzheimer disease. Discreetly entering the back of the room, the facility's director brought in a resident named Hazel, who did not want to stay seated in her wheelchair. Because Hazel was at risk for falling, it was apparent that the wheelchair was a safety precaution, so one of the student caregivers was asked to care for her during our class time. The caregiver stationed herself next to the resident, and the class discussion resumed.

It wasn't long before Hazel was out of her wheelchair and trying to escape from us, however. The student caregiver would get Hazel seated in her wheelchair only to find her a few seconds later scrambling back to her feet. While we clearly needed to divert her attention from trying to leave her wheelchair, she was obviously on some sort of mission. I decided to put into practice a technique that I had recently learned from Laura Wayman's caregiver training.

I started by introducing myself to Hazel, and then I calmly and politely asked her where she was going. She explained that she had to leave because she wanted to start her new business.

With those words, she had given me the opportunity to enter into her dementia world and demonstrate to the class the affirmative response method of communication. I shared with Hazel that we were holding a meeting regarding new businesses and would like to have her sit down and join us. Immediately—and with great enthusiasm—she sat back down into her wheelchair, and we were off to a great start!

With the rest of the class sitting with us, I asked Hazel about her upcoming entrepreneurial venture. She told us that she wanted to open a baby store to supply products to her clients. I involved the class in Hazel's dementia wonderland by guiding the students to discuss what might be stocked in a store like the one Hazel had in mind and how she might price the items. While giving these affirmative responses to Hazel, I continued teaching. I used this opportunity to demonstrate how important it is to get to know the residents they care for, and how much they need to relate to the residents' worlds. It was exciting to see how well the principles I had learned from Laura really worked.

My encounter with Hazel reminded me of a very important lesson. The main focus of providing care for the elderly, especially those who have dementia, is not about my agenda (like teaching a class), wanting someone like Hazel to sit back down in her wheelchair, or even my feelings. The focus is on the needs of the elderly person in front of me. The interaction with Hazel reinforced the idea that if I am going to be able to respond to the immediate needs of a person who has dementia, I must be willing to enter into his or her world attentively, respectfully, and without argument. Most importantly, I must treat each person with genuine loving care.

CHAPTER TEN

Lucy and Betty

Thinking Outside the Box

It came as a shock to the family when Grandma Lucy was diagnosed with Alzheimer's. The 87-year-old was always so bright and loved to be involved in her children's lives, spending hours with them and the grandchildren whenever possible. She never tired of sharing remarkable stories from her rich, long history. She was an attractive lady, taking immense pride in her appearance, even wearing matching shoes with every outfit.

But Lucy began to struggle emotionally. She also suffered the common losses of dementia—short-term memory malfunction and a breakdown in information processing. Her diabetes brought on major health complications. Finally, the family had to make the tough decision to place her in a memory care facility.

A mere two weeks after Lucy had settled in and was apparently making a smooth transition into her new home, the diabetes caused circulatory failure in her legs and set off a dramatic chain of events. Everything culminated in the unfortunate medical necessity to amputate both of her legs below the knee. After a long hospital stay and a brief time in rehabilitation, she was back "home" in the memory care facility—now in a wheelchair. But this time she did not make the transition smoothly.

Lucy returned with a disturbing behavior that was puzzling to her family, the staff, and the other residents. She would spend her days rolling around in her wheelchair from one resident to another, shaking her finger and yelling that they had stolen her shoes. Lucy would call out for the staff to "get her shoes back from that thief," angrily accusing everyone in her path. The staff would quietly assure her that no one had stolen her shoes and would attempt to bring her into reality by gently reminding her of the necessary but heartbreaking surgery and loss of her legs. This approach only escalated her paranoia, emotional distress, and anger. There seemed to be no way to calm or comfort her.

The staff and family consulted me for advice. After talking with Lucy's family about her past and the most recent events, I asked the daughter to tell me about Lucy's favorite pair of shoes.

Her daughter said, "Mom had so many pairs of shoes that it's hard to know which ones were her favorites. She did have a beautiful pair of red satin pumps; they were very stylish in her day, and she would often wear them to church or on special occasions. She even asked for them right after she moved here, before her surgery, but we did not want her wearing them because they have a very tall heel, and she could have easily taken a bad fall."

I asked the daughter if she would bring that pair of shoes to her mother. She looked bewildered and said they were packed away, but she would. When she brought in the shoes the next day, we all stood back as she handed them to Lucy. What happened next brought tears to our eyes. Lucy's face lit up, and she got a big, bright smile reminiscent of a child's on Christmas morning. She stroked the shoes, turning them this way and that to view every inch. Then she put them in her lap and rolled off in her wheelchair to proudly flaunt them to the other residents. She did not seem to mind that she could not wear them, only exhibiting utter satisfaction as she carried them everywhere in her lap. That night, the staff placed them on her nightstand in plain view, and Lucy relaxed and went to sleep.

The next day and from then on, she continued to contentedly carry, display, and admire her beautiful red shoes.

⁂

Betty loved living independently. She was a private person, enjoying time for herself in her home of forty-seven years. She had raised her only child, a daughter, in that house and would pass the time tending to her lovely garden, full of prize-winning roses. She would also spend countless hours sitting in her front porch swing, keeping track of the comings and goings in her neighborhood. Alert and curious, she would hear all, see all, and delight in telling all to her daughter whenever she would visit, passing along the gossip of the day about her neighbors.

That is, until she developed dementia. As Betty's abilities decreased, she needed more and more help with day-to-day tasks in her home. Betty's daughter lived only a few minutes away and recognized that she needed to balance the losses her mother was experiencing with her remaining abilities. The goal was to allow Betty to function independently and to enjoy living in her home as long as possible. She would watch her mother closely and step in and assist with care only when she truly needed help.

One of the difficult challenges the daughter had to face was letting Betty know it was no longer wise for her to drive. Betty's eyesight had deteriorated significantly, and her reaction times had slowed. She was not a safe driver. Her daughter now provided all of the transportation, organizing errands and shopping trips around her own work schedule so that Betty could keep her doctors' appointments, excursions to the beauty salon, luncheons with her friends, and grocery or shopping trips every week. This routine also gave the daughter an excuse to visit regularly, check on Betty's nutrition and medication needs, and help out with small chores and daily tasks.

But as the dementia progressed, Betty became more and more resistant to getting up and out of the house on time, especially for her appointments. On those days, the daughter would arrive in the morning a couple of hours before the appointment and find Betty still in bed.

"Time to get up, Mom!" the daughter would cheerfully exclaim, "Today you have an appointment with Dr. Smith at ten o'clock. I'm here early to help you get ready. I'll go start the shower while you get up."

Betty would sit up drowsily, look around and say, "Where do we have to go today?"

The daughter would say it again, "Today you have an appointment with Dr. Smith at ten o'clock. Rise and shine!"

Betty would lie back down and say, "I didn't sleep at all last night. Could we go another day?"

Already the daughter could feel the recurring frustration brewing. She had reminded her mother about this necessary appointment at dinnertime the day before. But the predictable and tedious routine was happening anyway. It was getting more and more difficult for the daughter to disguise her emotions, and her negative feelings showed through in her facial expressions and demeanor.

Betty was picking up on the frustrations but could not remember asking the questions and repeating herself, so she had no way to understand why her daughter was upset. It was all very confusing. With great concern and hesitation, she asked her daughter again, "Where are we going?"

With all her might the daughter attempted to stay calm: "You have a doctor's appointment in an hour. We have to hurry to get there in time."

I listened to the daughter explain the frustrating circumstances. She felt like a terrible daughter and caregiver for getting so annoyed with her sweet mother. She said that she knew her mother could not remember, but it was still so difficult to keep reminding her every five minutes without going absolutely batty. And it felt like the harder she pushed Betty to cooperate and hurry, the slower and more resistant Betty became.

After getting to know Betty and her past likes and dislikes, I worked with her daughter to come up with a new approach. Happily, it worked like a charm. By reframing her approach only slightly, the daughter received the gift of an affirmative response. An added bonus was that the whole experience became meaningful and fun instead of tiresome and repetitive.

This is how it went: "Good morning, Mom, time to get up. I'm here to take you to your doctor appointment at ten o'clock. How did you sleep?"

Betty replied as she usually did, "I didn't sleep at all. Could we reschedule for another day?"

"No, Mom, but we can get you back here mid-morning to rest after the appointment. I'll go get the water started for your shower, but first I want to tell you a secret about your neighbor, Mrs. Jones." The daughter launched into a juicy story she made up about one of her mother's neighbors and then said, "Come get into the shower, and I'll tell you the rest."

Betty's eyes lit up, and her face was bright with interest. She stepped into the bathroom and listened intently to the "gossip" that her daughter conveyed. She was even cheerfully cooperative as she dressed, and her new, accommodating manner continued all the way through breakfast, the drive to the doctor's, the wait at the doctor's office, and the trip home.

As her daughter related the "gossip," Betty provided appropriate commentary: "Oh my goodness," "I'm shocked," and "I can't imagine!" The daughter reported that it was the best time she'd had with her mother in a long while! And from then on, this approach worked like magic!

Lessons Learned

The techniques employed with Lucy and Betty are called *creative interventions*. A creative intervention involves simply finding a clever way to meet the specific needs of a person who has dementia. Lucy wanted to hold her bright red shoes, and Betty loved gossip.

In developing your own creative interventions, you will find they work best if you have the opportunity to research and collect information from the individual's past. Each person with dementia has a unique and long history of joys, sorrows, pleasure, and pain. Tapping into the significance of historical events that make the individual feel loved, secure, valued, or safe will usually bring those feelings to the present time and allow you to share in the origins of the feelings attached to a memory. The better you come to understand the person for whom you are caring, the better able you will be to provide his or her care.

Alzheimer disease and other forms of dementia progress over time, affecting how the person functions on a day-to-day basis. As you learn about the changes the disease causes, you will develop realistic expectations of the person's abilities.

In the early stages, ask your loved one or client how you can help him or her stay independent and maintain a sense of control. It is best to encourage independence as much as possible, since doing so will reduce the burden on you and on the person for whom you are caring. As the dementia begins to hinder the person's memory and abilities, he or she will find it beneficial to contribute to self-care, even if it is in a small way.

To a point, independence boils down to the old saw: use it or lose it! Of course, later in the disease the person may well not be able to participate in his or her own self-care.

Perceptions and Approaches

A common tip from experienced caregivers is to *learn to be patient.* Granted, this is not always easy, but it will pay off in rich rewards. Do not rush people who have dementia. Give them plenty of time. Although it is often faster and easier to do things for other people rather than wait as they perform tasks for themselves, allowing them to complete basic tasks gives them a sense of value and helps them to feel proud of even the simplest accomplishments.

Above all, be sure to continue your favorite activities together: Listen to music. Take a walk. Talk about your favorite shoes. "Gossip" about the usual suspects. Focus on the person's talents and abilities. Look for common interests and use them to establish communication connections.

No matter how the disease affects the individual, it is important to treat him or her with dignity and respect. Although certain abilities will be lost, the person's emotions and feelings will remain, as will the need for companionship and belonging. To add to the person's quality of life and help him or her maintain a unique identity, provide activities and interactions that bring a sense of joy and celebration.

Never lose sight of the person who was there before the dementia.

CHAPTER ELEVEN

Edna

You're Just Imagining Things

🌿 🌿 🌿

One afternoon a middle-aged woman named Sue called the home care company that I was managing. Sue was her Aunt Edna's closest kin, but she lived several hours away from her aunt. When I picked up the crisis line, Sue explained the situation in a panicked voice: "Aunt Edna lives alone in a large house and has been doing okay until recently. Now I'm worried because this morning she called me and said I had to come to her house right now and get the clowns out of her living room."

You can imagine how Aunt Edna's plea sounded to her niece. Apparently, these "clowns" had kept Edna up all night, telling her they had come for the clothes she had taken from them. They would not leave her alone, and Edna was very afraid. The niece wanted to know if our company could provide a caregiver to stay with Edna and make sure there were no "clowns" who were causing this torment.

She explained, "Edna is threatening to call 911 to get the police to take out the clowns. There are no neighbors nearby that I can call on, so can I hire someone from your company to sit with her until I get there?"

I told the alarmed niece that I could do an emergency assessment within the hour and find out more about the situation. Then I would call her back and let her know if we could get a caregiver to help out until the family could make other arrangements.

When I arrived at Edna's house, she greeted me warmly at the door and immediately let me inside. I explained to Edna that I had experience in dealing with clowns, as well as other foolish visitors, and that in the past I had been successful in getting similar folk to leave the premises. Edna looked at me with incredible relief. "Last week I called the police," she sighed, "and they simply told me there were no clowns. They left me alone with them."

She was thankful that I believed her and that I wanted to do something to solve the problem. I use open-ended questions to help people with dementia guide me through their wonderland, which helps me understand their perception and reality. It is important to begin each question with "who?" "what?" "where?" "when?" or "how?"

"Where are these annoying clowns?" I asked her. Edna pointed to a large sofa. Sighing with frustration at my lack of awareness, she said, "All three of them are right there, as you can plainly see." I watched her face and realized that she could indeed see clowns sitting right there in front of us. To her, they were very real.

So I walked over to the sofa where the "clowns" were camped out and said in a firm and confident tone: "What are you here for? I need to ask you to leave now!"

Edna piped in with a condescending tone in my direction, "They want their clothes back. I already told everyone that."

Continuing to face the clowns, I asked Edna, "Where are these clothes?"

Edna led me down the hall to her bedroom and her overstuffed clothes closet. I asked her to hand me the items of clothing that she believed were the ones the clowns were asking for. Without hesitation, she handed me several brightly colored items out of her closet. I asked her if this was all of them. Edna nodded, and I carried the clothes out to my car.

As I exited the house, I looked over my shoulder and said to the nonexistent clowns, "This is all of it. I will take you and the clothes back to where you belong, and you must never come here again and bother this nice lady." (The clowns were indeed "nonexistent" in my reality, but Edna's behavior showed they existed and were very "real" in her dementia wonderland.)

I put everything in my trunk and went back inside the house to let Edna know I would take care of this matter and that she had nothing to worry about. I also told her that I had a coworker who was coming right over to keep her company until her niece arrived. Edna seemed grateful and calm; resolving her problem had made her feel safe and secure.

The caregiver from our company arrived a few minutes later, and for several months she came to stay with Edna on a regular schedule, at the family's request. Edna never again claimed to see or be bothered by clowns. Our office quietly returned the brightly colored clothing back to Edna's closet without incident.

Lessons Learned

Unfortunately, as individuals struggle to cope with dementia, paranoia like Edna's is not uncommon. People with dementia may have misperceptions or hallucinations about family members, old friends, and strangers. In most cases, this is just a phase that eventually subsides, but there is no way to predict how long these symptoms will last. The severity of the symptoms can depend on the type of dementia.

The resulting behaviors are especially related to a loss of control. As people with dementia come to rely on others for assistance, they may feel as if the caregivers are taking over their lives or even robbing them. And as the dementia progresses, they often lose the ability to recognize that they themselves might be to blame for missing items. For example, they might store some valuables away to protect the items from theft and then forget where they hid them. It would then seem to them that the misplaced items must have been stolen, and they will often accuse the people closest to them of stealing the items.

If a person with dementia still lives in his or her own home, the most likely target of the accusations will be the family or professional in-home caregiver—or possibly a housekeeper or landscaper. In a care facility, such as an assisted living or memory care community, the main target generally will be the care staff, other residents, or even visitors. You may hear statements such as these:

- "A man came here and he took my jewelry."
- "That woman stole my scarves, but she says she didn't take them."

Instead of reacting to these behaviors, coping with and managing them is the key to making the person feel safe and supported. Imagine what it would be like if you suspected you were being followed home by a strange car one evening, thought you had been receiving odd or threatening phone calls, or believed you saw someone hiding outside your bedroom window. Now imagine that you shared your fears with your family and friends, and that even though you were genuinely scared, they calmly dismissed your anxiety as foolishness. How would this make you feel?

Perceptions and Approaches

As noted in earlier chapters, it is best not to argue with a confused person. Disagreeing may only escalate and fan the fires of anger, anxiety, paranoia, and fear. If you cannot win the battle, change the war. No matter how outlandish the claim or accusation, listen and proceed as though you believe everything the person with dementia is saying. Plan to take action that will give the person a sense of relief. The most frustrating response she can get from you is an argument to try to convince her that the situation is not real. Although in this instance it was helpful for me to ask Edna questions, because she still could process this information and give me answers, keep in mind that as the dementia progresses, it becomes more and more difficult for the person to respond. A dementia-aware caregiver uses fewer questions and gives fewer options and instead takes positive action and makes simple statements. The more you "think" for people with dementia, the kinder and more supportive you are in their eyes. Short and sweet, less is best, fewer words and more action. Agree, agree, and agree some more! This change in your care approach as you become more and more dementia-aware will bring you much relief, as well as help the one you are caring for experience more moments of calmness and peace.

This is a big change in how we have always communicated with adults, so it takes practice! I even have to remind myself to ask less and do more, as this is a core component of dementia-aware communication. For example, when you first greet someone you often ask, "How are you?" You expect a common response such as "Fine, how are you?" I have observed how this ordinary and simple question can make the person with dementia uncomfortable, stopping them in their tracks as they struggle to process an answer. When I began to notice this was causing some difficulties, I changed this customary greeting to a positive statement such as, "You look great today!" or "It is so nice to meet you!" The change in their response was remarkable, so much more relaxed and less confused. I now make it a habit to communicate more and more often in this manner, starting from the first moment I spend with the person who has dementia symptoms.

Many of the things that people with dementia do are attempts to empower themselves by hanging on to the remaining elements of control and choice they still possess. As we go through life, we suffer diminishing control over many things. These losses put dents in our emotional armor, especially if they are caused by dementia. Examples include loss of

- memory
- knowing where you are and who other people are
- physical health
- relationships
- independence, such as the ability to drive or to take care of personal finances
- the ability to care for the basic needs of daily living, such as bathing, eating, grooming, toileting, walking, or even standing up

It is vital to allow people to retain a sense of control as far as you and they are able:

- If Mom feels secure when she has a credit card and checkbook (even though the accounts are closed), then let her have them, even though you are now in charge of the finances.

- If Dad keeps claiming that someone is poisoning his food, perhaps what he means is that the food tastes very different. He may fear that the food is somehow a cause of his confusion and loss.

Given all of the other losses that persons with dementia may be experiencing, the last thing they want to feel is that they have lost their grip on reality. When people with dementia insist that the people around them affirm their perception of the world, they are actually asking for help in framing their own worlds. By providing validation, you will help to make everything else seem less confusing to them, even if the relief is only temporary. Your affirmation provides a brief respite, allowing the person with dementia to rest his or her mind in the midst of what must feel like constant chaos.

Remember that each situation and scenario is very real and true to your loved one or client in his or her wonderland. It must be very frightening to experience events that seem so real and then not receive validation from others. As you listen to and focus on every complaint, accusation, or angry outburst, try to allow yourself to be open to what is being said. Being open will let you develop steps to solve the person's challenges, just as you would tackle real problems. Be a detective and discover the who, what, when, where, and how of each situation. Handling your loved one or client's issues is yet another way to bridge the gap between the two of you and enter into the dementia wonderland. And if helping "get the clowns out of the house" will bring the person with dementia to a place of calm, then get creative and do what it takes.

The restlessness and anxiety that accompanies the person with dementia on a daily basis can be overwhelming. As noted in earlier chapters, there is always an underlying reason for the person's behavior—generally a feeling or memory from the past that is causing confusion, fear, anger, paranoia, or aggressiveness in the present. Sometimes the person may be searching for someone or something, not even knowing who or what it is she is looking for. Worst of all, the person with dementia does not know how to resolve or calm the constant sense of tension and frustration. Having the caregiver believe what the person is saying may be the only key to peace and serenity.

As you approach each situation with an open mind, also consider the possibility that a person's behavior may not be totally rooted in dementia. For example, the paranoia caused by dementia may be exacerbated by sensory impairment.

I once heard a story of an elderly man who continually told his family that the president of the United States came to visit him. The family would upset this gentleman by arguing with him that this was not possible. Then one day the son walked into his father's room when the presidential debates were on TV. The father had impaired vision and was hard of hearing, and the TV was blaring in the background. The gentleman was not hallucinating or telling stories; he had poor eyesight and difficulty distinguishing between what was real and what he was hearing on the television. He truly believed the president was in the room with him.

Throughout the dementia journey, all you can do is your best as you face the challenging role of caring for your loved one or client. You may be able to count up the many things that you feel you have done wrong, but the fact is that we are all human and make mistakes. Take time to find a little magic in each day and celebrate the small wins along the journey.

When your loved one or client is affected by dementia-related paranoia, he or she may make some very hurtful accusations. Even though you are making tremendous sacrifices to take care of her, she may angrily look you straight in the eye and say things like, "You stole my purse! I know it was you!" These kinds of comments hurt, and they may be devastating, even triggering your own past wounds and conflicts. If you are a professional caregiver, there may be the added fear of losing your job when the person with dementia makes accusations of theft. In these instances, be sure to communicate with your manager or supervisor. Additionally, you may need to have a meeting with the person's family to discuss the situation. Whether you are a professional caregiver or a lay caregiver, let these situations be powerful reminders of your own need for self-care.

As frequently as possible, look for easy ways to lighten your load. Lock the bathroom door and soak in a bubble bath. Get together with your friends and play cards. Take a walk or read a book. Watch the latest ballgame or a comforting movie. Choose your favorite relaxing activity. You need to have a place where you can remove stress and emotionally vent.

In addition to practicing these quick fixes, schedule time for long-term stress management and maintenance. Longer-term stress busters can include attending regular caregiver support groups (the local chapter of the Alzheimer's Association can provide lists of support groups in your area), seeing a counselor who is experienced in caregiver stress issues, or learning meditation or progressive relaxation exercises. There are also wonderful training programs that are specific to stress management and that are suited to both family caregivers and healthcare professionals.

One such program that is currently receiving rave reviews is called HeartMath. HeartMath training programs, coaching, publications, licensing programs, and innovative technology may help people live more rewarding and healthy lives—personally and professionally. I have not tried these training programs myself and mention them only as an example of the kinds of programs that are being developed.

Early in my own dementia care journey, I worked alongside a local medical hypnotherapist who professionally recorded relaxation and mood-enhancing CDs. These CDs contained soothing music that helped me reduce my own stress and provided a calming environment for the people with dementia whom I was working with as well. Many CDs with calming music and words are available through bookstores, libraries, and online.

Some in-home care providers and dementia care facilities use a program called Snoezelen Therapy, which is designed to assist in calming people with dementia who are agitated. Snoezelen Therapy utilizes a "relaxation room" that consists of fiber-optic lighting fixtures, aromatherapy, soft and changing environmental mood lighting, comfortable seating, and relaxing sounds and music. By engaging as many senses as possible, this atmosphere may create a sense of safety and security. Again, I have not tried this program with my clients.

Whether you are a family or professional caregiver, during these tough days and moments I encourage you to do whatever it takes to manage your stress level. This includes the time-honored practice of asking for assistance. Attending a support group will help you find out what other caregivers have done to cope with the bizarre stories, unfounded accusations, and paranoia that the person with dementia may exhibit. To further educate yourself, attend an educational conference, seminar, or workshop. It is imperative that you protect and safeguard yourself from the potential negative impacts of this disease.

CHAPTER TWELVE

Margie

If You Keep Doing What You Are Doing . . .

The daughter of a German woman and a US soldier, Margie grew up in postwar Germany. We can only imagine what her childhood was like. We do know that she and her family spent a year in a tuberculosis ward. Her father, a military cook, was often away, and Margie ended up caring for her mother, who suffered from depression, as well as for her sister, who was targeted by bullies at school because she was deaf (a result of meningitis). Although Margie was mentally and physically abused by her mother and was often battered in scuffles while defending her sister, she maintained a positive outlook on life. Eventually, her family moved to America.

Years later, in 1968, Margie met Pete, a sailor based at an air station in Maine. The following year, they were married. Margie and Pete enjoyed an amazing marriage and had one child, Jennifer. Eventually they moved to California and ended up in the foothills above Sacramento.

In 2007, Pete began noticing worrisome signs in his wife. Though she was still relatively young to be diagnosed with dementia, she had increasingly noticeable short-term memory loss and struggled to recall things that had never been a problem in the past. Both of Margie's parents had died of Alzheimer disease, so Pete and Margie were familiar with the symptoms. Pete was proactive and consulted with their family physician. Margie was diagnosed with early-onset Alzheimer disease.

This was the beginning of a long and difficult downward spiral. In the months following the diagnosis, Margie got confused and turned the wrong direction at the end of their driveway, backing into a tree. She would also get lost driving to familiar places within a short distance of home.

To make matters worse, she began to have frequent bouts of anxiety and paranoia, with the result that she wandered away from home. Several times, Pete was forced to ask the local police for help in bringing her back safely. On Margie's fifty-eighth birthday, she went to church with her husband and wept uncontrollably throughout the entire sermon. Afterward, to Pete's dismay, she refused to get in the car. Extremely agitated, she started walking, and Pete followed her closely in the car. Then she waved down a passing car and got in, driving off with perfect strangers. Fortunately, they drove her right back to church. Pete followed, but she again refused to get into his car.

From there she took off on foot and disappeared. It was the police who found her standing in front of a nearby Catholic church. Margie remained adamant about not leaving with Pete, so he called their daughter, and Margie agreed to go home with Jennifer for the time being. Pete was so shaken by the unfortunate situation that he had to be admitted to the hospital for extremely high blood pressure. He was experiencing the stress-related physical strain of caregiving for a memory-challenged adult. Pete came to the painful realization that he would have to get Margie additional care from another source.

Margie was placed in a memory care environment, but she did not adjust well. After a brief hospital stay, she was placed in a skilled nursing facility. But this particular institution was not proficient in managing the type of dementia behaviors that Margie exhibited, including anger, combativeness, and anxiety. The situation went from bad to worse.

When the staff called Pete to discuss his wife's severe behavioral problems, Pete contacted me for help. He explained that she had pushed, hit, and kicked a male caregiver who had tried to assist her with a shower. And this was not the only incident. When she was acting out in her fear and anger, she would even threaten other residents.

In what would become a cycle, after an episode of combative behavior the staff would send Margie to a hospital for a mental health assessment, and the hospital would send her back—over and over.

Unfortunately, this type of situation is common in facilities that do not properly train staff with the communication tools to gently and lovingly redirect the person with dementia. I agreed to spend a few hours with Margie at the facility. My plan was to then approach the facility staff with some training solutions so they could more successfully manage Margie's agitation and aggression.

When I arrived, Margie was in the activity room with a group that was playing a game. She sat at the table with the other residents but was not engaged at all. After a few minutes, she stood up. Most of her waking time was spent walking around and around the hallways. In fact, she slept very little and rarely sat still.

Her daughter, Jennifer, introduced me to Margie as a friend of hers. Pete was also there and gave Margie a kiss on the cheek. She smiled at both of them and said hello to me. We chatted as we walked together and sat for a few minutes in the lobby. It was apparent that Margie felt uncomfortable sitting for any length of time. Pete explained that she had back pain, and I wondered if this was one of the reasons she was constantly on the move. After forty-five minutes of visiting and walking, I recognized it was time for a staff member to change Margie. She was incontinent and needed to be cleaned up. As we passed the nurse's station, I discreetly requested the change. The male nurse asked me to take her to her room so he could send someone to take care of her personal needs.

Her room was long and narrow, with three beds and curtains to section off each bed area for privacy; hers was at the very back. As we entered, Margie's calm and pleasant demeanor instantly changed to suspicion—to that of a frightened victim. She became nervous and looked at me with sudden distrust. As I turned to go back out into the hallway, two male caregivers marched in to change Margie.

They moved with determination toward her and pulled the privacy curtain. In less than two minutes, Margie came bursting into the hall with her pants unzipped and her face bright red with rage. She was screaming and cursing, vowing that she would never go back there. She made her way to the nurse's counter, picked up a pile of books and a book stand, and pitched them at the nurse behind the counter. Pete and I came up beside her and, as calmly as we could, talked to her and stroked her arms. This was a method that always worked for Pete when he needed to calm her from an agitated state. Jennifer was then able to walk her down the hall and further quiet her.

I asked the nurse in charge if they had female staff available to change Margie, since it was obvious that she was very frightened by the male care providers. I was told that they were unable to fulfill that kind of request due to difficulty scheduling enough female nurses to cover every shift. Moreover, they needed to send caregivers strong enough to "hold her down to change her." Pete, Jennifer, and I were astonished. We reminded the nurse that Margie had not exhibited aggression in the hospital or with female care providers.

However, we were ultimately met with a refusal to modify the approach. The saddest part of this story is that after the next time Margie was taken to the hospital, the nursing facility refused to take her back, stating that they could not manage her care and that her behavior was too difficult for them to handle.

It has been said that insanity is doing the same thing over and over and expecting a different result. In this instance, the facility staff's inflexibility made it impossible for them to care for Margie adequately.

Lessons Learned

Research is showing that some relatively basic interventions that do not involve pharmaceuticals can be used to ease behaviors. A simplified approach to managing agitation can be summed up as "modify the environment, modify the behavior, and medicate as a last resort." While most of this research was conducted in residential facilities and nursing homes, family caregivers can follow the same principles.

In our professional caregiving training sessions, we always tell the care providers, "If you keep doing what you are doing, you will keep getting what you are getting." And if what you are getting is not an *affirmative response,* try a different approach.

All types of behavior are forms of communication. When a person with dementia acts out, he or she is trying to tell you something. Agitation is often the result of the inability to deal with stress, pain, or fatigue. The key is to identify whether the behavior is related to a specific event or whether it stems from a sudden or unusual environmental stimulation that causes an emotional outburst and then escalates into a combative flare-up:

- An *event-related cause* could be an unpleasant situation involving necessary care, such as when a caregiver attempts to clean the person up after an incontinence-related accident. The care receiver may strongly feel that his or her privacy is being invaded by a stranger. The event may even bring up memories from an abusive past event.
- *Environmental stimulation* that causes agitation could involve, for example, moving the person with dementia from their home into a hospital-like skilled nursing facility. It may be that the person feels bereaved because he or she associates the hospital setting with a memory of the loss of a loved one.

Either of these kinds of memory stimulations—which are usually innocent—can trigger unpleasant, seemingly bizarre, or even dangerous actions on the part of the person with dementia.

Take note of patterns and subtle clues that tension is mounting. The more proactive you are in redirecting the behavior before anxiety escalates, the more successful the redirection will be. Avoid telling people with dementia "no" or "you can't" or trying to physically prevent them from going somewhere or doing something. This could be perceived as aggression, and they will feel they must forcefully protect themselves. The tendency toward aggressive behavior often increases at the end of the day as stress and fatigue build.

Perceptions and Approaches

What are some ways to deal with agitation?

I have enjoyed great success using music with which the person with dementia is familiar. Playing calming music or the person's favorite type of music can lead to a decrease in agitation. Use this tool before and during meals, since it can increase food and fluid consumption. When relaxing and calming music is used during bathing, it can make the person with dementia less resistant to personal care. Use the music familiar to those growing up in the thirties, forties, and fifties. Try everything from soothing classical music to hymns and spirituals or big band tunes.

Light exercise each day can also help to maintain function of limbs and decrease problem behaviors. Going for a walk—preferably one to two hours before dinner—several times each week may help reduce pent-up agitation in a healthy, productive way, as well as stimulate the appetite. And besides, exercise is good for *you*, the caregiver, too.

Activities that include social interaction are also helpful. Sometimes large groups and many strangers are not well received, but a companion or volunteer who consistently spends one-on-one time with your loved one or client is usually welcome.

Additionally, never lose sight of the person who was there before the dementia. Activities that reflect your loved one's previous life or career are very effective. And everyone can derive pleasure from the simplest activities. You can reminisce, converse, or sing together.

Above all, a serene approach *from the caregiver* is the magical key to successfully managing agitation. The person with dementia is ultra-sensitive to your moods and feelings and will mirror back whatever is felt from the person providing care. So check your anxiety, agitation, and stress at the door before you spend time with a person with dementia.

CHAPTER THIRTEEN

Harry

It's Bath Night!

Born and raised in Denver, I grew up in the beautiful state of Colorado. My father's father, Harry William, who was born in England, immigrated to the United States at the young age of 13. He came through Ellis Island, worked hard, married, and raised two children, one of whom was my father, Jack. When Harry retired, he built a small log cabin in the picturesque village of Red Feather Lakes in the Colorado Rockies.

I was the youngest of five siblings, and our family also had many foster children. Every summer, we would all spend several weeks at Grandpa Harry's cabin. The mountain slopes provided ample space to run, climb rocks, fish, catch frogs, and dig for worms. We would also ride the wooden horses that Grandpa had built out of logs, have fun in the playhouse he had built with his own hands, and make popcorn in the cabin's fireplace.

The cabin had no running water or electricity and the fireplace was effectively the central heating unit. When we needed water, Grandpa Harry would haul it from the well. Needless to say, we children managed to get rather dirty while playing in our mountain paradise. Now that I think about it, we probably did not smell particularly good, either.

However, Grandpa Harry had a once-a-week routine for cleaning up that he had brought with him from his younger days. When we visited him, we were treated to the same time-honored tradition of the Saturday night bath. Grandpa would heat up the bath water on the wood-burning stove in the kitchen, then pour the hot water into the big aluminum tub. We all took turns, oldest first, in the progressively dirtier and colder water.

Since I was the youngest, I always got the coldest and dirtiest water! At the time I didn't mind, but as an adult, I still remember the cool water and not being able to see the bottom of the tub through all the grime from my older siblings. There was not a shower or a bathtub with running water in sight, and I am positive that if we had asked Grandpa about taking a shower, he would have looked at us as if we were speaking a foreign language.

Taking showers, especially seven days a week, is a tradition that belongs to later generations. In my grandfather's day, water was a precious commodity and bathing was a major production: clean water had to be hauled in and heated and dirty water had to be hauled out. Baths happened once a week. Daily cleaning-up consisted of a sponge bath. This "bird bath," as my mother called it, involved a bar of soap, cold water, and a clean rag or sponge.

Lessons Learned

Many people who have dementia resist personal care tasks like bathing. When caregivers ask me to help them overcome this reluctance, they often tell me the same story: they ask the care recipient whether he or she wants to take a shower, and the response is a firm "No." "I just took one," he might say, or "It's not time yet." Or the person might stare blankly, as if she doesn't understand the question. Once I was providing care for a family friend whose father reacted to bathing by crying in the shower. He repeated over and over that it was too hot or too cold and pleaded with me to stop or to hurry up and finish. It was an unpleasant experience for both of us. Sometimes the topic of showering obviously makes the person who has dementia feel afraid, a response that makes me wonder why the person is having such an extreme reaction to a common daily task.

To solve this mystery, we must remember that people who have dementia travel back into their pasts, retrieving old memories and feelings. They tend to seek those memories that make them feel secure, safe, and happy. The language of dementia and each person's unique dialect come from long-ago traditions and events. They also rely on all five senses: sight, hearing, smell, taste, and touch.

Bearing this in mind, we can explore whether the word *shower* means the same thing to the person who has dementia as the word *bath*. What memories might be brought to mind by a shower? Water hitting him in the face, for example? Or might a bath bring to mind easing her toes into the water to test its temperature? Was the room where he bathed as a child a cold, tiny space with glaring white tiles and bright lights, or was it a lantern-lit kitchen in a farmhouse warmed by a cozy fire? Were the sounds of bathing harsh and echoing, or were they the familiar voices of family members? Was their family very private, or were others allowed to wash and touch sensitive parts of their nude bodies?

Now imagine what it would be like to experience a shower in an unfamiliar place with strange people around you.

Perceptions and Approaches

It's no wonder that caregivers frequently face resistance to the common task of bathing. A sensitive approach may make all the difference. When your loved one or client resists letting you help him or her with a shower, avoid saying the word *shower* or *asking questions*. Instead, try simple and positive action statements:

- "It's time to clean up now."
- "Let's go take our bath before the water gets too cold and dirty."
- "I am so hot; a cool bath would make me feel better. I'm going that way, so come and give me a hand getting the bath ready."
- "A warm bath sounds so good. It would warm you down to your bones."
- "Your daughter called and said she is on her way to take you to _____ [the doctor's office, lunch, etc.]." Use whatever topic might motivate this person to get ready.

- "It's Saturday. Time for bath night!" Draw on the person's past routine, if you know what it was. Use terms that are understandable within the person's dialect of dementia.
- "I picked up your favorite lavender-scented soap. You smell so good when you use it. Let's go use some right now."

If the approach is not working now, come back and try again at a time when he or she is more likely to be cooperative. If Mrs. Smith is not a morning person, approach her in the afternoon when she is in a better mood.

Bathing an elderly person who has dementia in a traditional bathtub is difficult and dangerous, so you may want to give the person a shower, even though you call the undertaking a "bath." You need to make the routine as familiar as possible, however. If there is a shower bench, have the person sit down; this is generally safer anyway. Use a handheld adjustable showerhead. It can be startling for anyone to be suddenly hit in the face by running water, so start by washing the feet and work your way up. Move slowly and with confident purpose. Talk in a quiet and reassuring tone. If you are nervous or rushed, the person will pick up on it and feel the same way.

Here are some more tips to make each bathing experience more peaceful and cooperative:

- Make sure the setting is quiet and private, with adequate but not overly glaring lights. A stark or bright light can feel cold and institutional. Honor the need for modesty; hold up a towel or undress and redress the person as you go. It is always appreciated if you provide assistance while keeping the person's dignity in mind.
- Be prepared. Have everything that is needed at hand: soap, towels, brush, etc. If you get the person ready and in a cooperative mood for bathing, you do not want to miss the window of opportunity because you have to go fetch a towel. Furthermore, it is not safe to leave the person alone, especially if he or she is wet and soapy.
- Give instructions *one* at a time. Do not rush the task. Keep in mind that the person's ability to process information has

been slowed and interrupted by the dementia, so keep
everything simple.

- Demonstrate the task at hand. A demonstration sometimes
  prompts the individual to begin the task himself or herself.
  For example, the person may begin to comb his or her own
  hair by watching you comb yours. Remember to always allow
  the person to do whatever he or she can. Do not focus on
  what is no longer within the person's abilities; encourage the
  person to do what he or she is capable of. Even a small sense
  of accomplishment feels good.

- Consider your own attitude and appearance. What is important? If it turns out that your loved one or client can tolerate
  a shower only once or twice a week—with a sponge bath
  every day in between—consider this a small compromise in
  the whole scheme of caregiving. If the person is not incontinent, the shower and sponge bath rotation usually provides
  adequate personal care. Most likely it will also become a
  familiar and comforting routine. As you take care of your
  own hygiene regularly, it sets a good example for the behavior you desire from your loved one or client. Even though
  people who have dementia may not be as aware of their own
  hygiene, they will still evaluate yours. It is not uncommon
  for ladies from prior generations to be critical of other women
  who venture out in public without full makeup and a fine
  hairdo. Older men who used to pride themselves on their
  fitness have no verbal filter and may tell people point-blank
  when they need to lose weight.

- Play soft music, preferably the style that is the person's favorite.
  When the person is in his or her "happy place" and enjoying
  music, he or she is more likely to be cooperative. Additionally, praise and compliments always help, just as noted by
  the old saying, "You can catch more flies with honey than
  you can with vinegar!"

- Finally, some caregivers have found that promising care
  recipients a bowl of ice cream can work wonders as an
  incentive.

You will probably encounter days when things go smoothly and other days when they do not. The person with dementia has mood swings like everyone else. Just stay on course and be willing to be flexible in your approaches. If bath time does not get done this morning, try the afternoon or tomorrow.

For more tips and strategies on successfully conquering the common struggle of bathing a person who has dementia, see the last chapter of this book, "The Dementia-Aware Guide to Caregiving," under "Challenges with Personal Hygiene." You may also want to read *Bathing without a Battle: Person-Directed Care of Individuals with Dementia*, by Ann Louise Barrick and coauthors. Like its popular predecessor, the second edition of *Bathing without a Battle* presents an individualized problem-solving approach to bathing and providing personal care for individuals with dementia. This edition includes historical material on bathing and substantially updates the section on special concerns, which includes pain, skin care, identifying the appropriate level of assistance, transfers, and the environment.

CHAPTER FOURTEEN

Rose, Edith, and Samuel

One Size Does Not Fit All

It was difficult for me to watch Samuel stand up and move from one place to another. His Parkinson's had made his previously strong and tall frame into what now resembled a tower of quivering and vibrating Jell-O. Every movement demanded mindful thought, and every step was a precarious prelude to another fall. The memory care staff would patiently allow Samuel to do as much as he could on his own, but even the simple act of sitting down would culminate in a hard thump into the wheelchair as his muscles would give out halfway down and send his large frame crashing into the seat. He was unable to sit up straight and his long frame leaned way over his knees, giving him only a limited view of the floor directly in front of him. Samuel would daily request his usual seat in the common area of the memory care community after the staff assisted him with all of the tasks necessary in the morning, assistance with dressing, shaving, brushing his teeth, etc. Samuel had taken up residence a few years before, as his Parkinson's had continued to take away the ability of his elderly wife to provide the increasingly demanding level of appropriate care for him at home. In order for myself, family, or the care staff to engage with Samuel, we had to sit on the floor directly in front of him as that was his limited view of the world. His Parkinsonian stiffness, constant tremors, and rigidness made it impossible for him to sit up and see what was going on beyond this limited visual scope. So, therefore, it was difficult for him to participate in activities, even though they were going on all around him. But he always insisted on sitting with the group, at least this was better than sitting alone in his room. That is, until one day I discovered a special way to help Samuel connect and engage!

On this particular afternoon, as the executive director of this memory care community, I was observing the scheduled group activity and although I was observing all of the residents, I was watching Samuel, Rose, and Edith in particular. The new activity leader of only two weeks, Mindy, had met with me that morning and shared some of her frustration with the challenges she was experiencing during group activities, specifically with three of our residents in memory care. Mindy felt that she was having some success engaging and providing activities that were enjoyable for most of the residents, however, the three she wanted to talk about, Rose, Edith, and Samuel, so far in her short tenure, had not shown the ability to connect and participate in a way that she felt was as meaningful as she had hoped.

I stopped by to observe for the afternoon and hopefully give some advice and strategies to overcome this often-common type of dementia challenge that comes with activities. Mindy was standing at the front of the common area, surrounded by residents sitting in a semi-circle, showing pictures of planes, trains, and automobiles of past eras. The majority of the residents were taking part with varying levels of interest and participation, some quietly watching, a couple catnapping, and a few even contributing to a spirited discussion. I always love to see and hear the residents as they reminisce and share the way important life events made them feel in the past, and how they can still benefit from the way many of these events can make them feel in the present. I smiled as Rose, one of our residents who had not been with us very long, and as Mindy had shared with me earlier, had not engaged up until now with this much excitement and clarity, suddenly began to participate and share. All of the staff and myself knew a bit about Rose's history. She had been a working professional woman at the time when most women were not a part of the outside workforce, and she was talking excitedly about the picture of the train that Mindy was holding up and discussing. Rose exclaimed, "That is the train I take to work every day. I catch it at 6:45 every morning at the station two blocks from my home. It drops me off six blocks from my office, and sometimes I have to walk in the bitter cold." You could see her shiver as she told us about her daily commute that included many blustery cold walks, and how, as she reminisced, she actually "felt the cold air."

I glanced over at Samuel and was troubled as I watched him attempt to look up and see the picture as he, to a certain degree, wanted to take interest in the picture and Rose's story. I kept thinking, "How can we help him experience meaning with his extreme physical limitations?" As Mindy moved to the next picture, I picked up the train picture and brought it to Samuel, sitting on the floor at his feet and right below his gaze. I said, "Here is the picture that Rose was talking about. She rode this train to work every day." I was a bit disheartened as Samuel briefly glanced at the picture but did not really show as much interest as I had wanted him to, in spite of my efforts to help him have the opportunity to engage.

The next picture Mindy held up for discussion was an older black-and-white photo of a silver commercial airliner with Pan Am painted on the side. As Mindy began to describe the picture, I saw Samuel begin to slightly straighten up in his chair, making a much bigger effort to see what he could only hear in his hunched over position. His interest was markedly increased as the detailed description was presented of this new photo, and he strained to see more. I could see that this was touching strong feelings deep down, something was stirring in him that literally made him attempt to "sit up and pay attention!" As I sat there on the floor in front of him, I said to Samuel, "I love to travel, and flying is my favorite. Tell me about your favorite airplane ride." What happened next made me want to jump for joy. Samuel slowly straightened in his chair, as much as he possibly could, and looked right into my eyes. He said, in a confident, almost defiant tone, "I was an airline pilot for Pan Am for thirty-five years, and I flew all over the world! I loved every flight!" There it was, what all of us as professionals look for—the gift of finding that unique gateway into the individual's dementia wonderland. These meaningful connections show us that the person is still there behind the horrific physical and cognitive losses of any cause of dementia, and it is so gratifying to share their feelings of value, accomplishment, and love that dementia-aware methods can help us together to experience. I jumped up, went to my office, and printed a pin on "badge" that said. "Talk to me about my thirty-five years as a Pan Am pilot." (A perfect example of a positive action statement—no questions!) Samuel eagerly agreed to wear his "badge," and I encouraged everyone, family, staff, and even visitors to sit with him and let him share his past feelings of accomplishment as a pilot. I was so pleased as I watched him smile and even sit up a little straighter in his chair (and demonstrate an example of an affirmative response).

Ah, but even though Samuel and Rose found meaning in a picture of a train and an airplane, there was still one other resident, Edith, that continued to show no signs of participating in this, or any of the other group activities that had been going on throughout the day. Just as there is no perfect one-size-fits-all in our overall dementia care approach and communication strategies, there is no one-size-fits-all that applies to dementia care activities. This is one of the biggest challenges we as professionals (and family members) encounter in dementia care, finding a way to connect and engage in a group setting, or even the one-on-one activities that family members are challenged with at home. Each individual with dementia symptoms struggles with different processing deficiencies and functional losses—loss of the ability to process what they see, what they hear, how to move—making each part of any activity challenging in part and as a whole. Because there is such specific loss for each person, there is simply no good cookie cutter approach to activities, or dementia care in general. Samuel had physical limitations along with cognitive decline, preventing him from actively participating in group discussions due to his limited vision and physical challenges. Rose had less limited ability physically but struggled to process information that she could see and hear, and could not always understand and utilize information that was not familiar or was new to her, as often is the case with dementia. So it was necessary to "think for her," to find something she could relate to and find comfortingly familiar from her unique past. Score two for Mindy and me, in a room of fifteen residents, all with different and distinct abilities and losses. However, even though most of these residents were able to participate to one degree or another in the majority of activities presented throughout the day, there were still the few residents who were not able to engage much or at all.

Edith was the third resident that Mindy and I had discussed earlier in the day, and in the more advanced stages of Alzheimer's, she was often restless and disengaged. She shuffled back and forth, not appearing to hear or see what was happening around her, often carrying on conversations with seemingly no one but herself. None of the group activities Mindy had tried seemed to hold her interest, as it was obvious that she could not process what she could see or any of what she heard. Yet Mindy and I continued to believe we could find something that would give her meaning, even if it was only momentary. As Edith passed by me, I joined her, walking with her down the hall. We passed one of the activity life stations, specifically the "Baby Station" that consisted of a crib, lifelike baby dolls, some infant clothing, and baby bottles. (Note: When we talk about "Life Stations," we are talking about the activity and engagement stations set up specifically for residents with dementia. These stations should be a main focus in dementia care communities, and allow residents space and engagement opportunities throughout the day.) I stopped and picked up the lifelike baby doll out of the crib in the "Baby Station" and, as I handed it to Edith, I said, "The baby is crying and wants you to hold her." (A great example of the success of using a "positive action statement" rather than succumbing to the usual way we have learned to communicate by asking a question: "Do you want to hold the baby?") Edith instinctively held out her hands and took the baby doll from me, held it close, and began to pat its back, muttering softly, "It's okay, don't cry." Then she turned and walked down the hallway, continuing to feel worth as she comforted the baby in her arms! Once again, a gift—for that moment the baby gave Edith momentary feelings of value and love, what we as humans crave and seek throughout all of our lives. Unfortunately, the loss of brain function and dementia symptoms interferes with Edith's ability to find these moments without our help.

Lessons Learned

"Life Stations" should replicate things that we see in normal, everyday life. Here are some great examples of life stations that you can bring to your community:

- Office Station with a desk, older model desk phone, typewriter, etc.
- Baby Station with a crib, baby dolls, baby clothes and blankets, and baby bottles.
- Kitchen Station with dishware, pots, pans, and a counter with mixing bowls and spoons.
- Teachers' Station with a chalkboard, desk, notebook, picture books, and coloring books.
- The Man Cave with sanding blocks, pieces of wood, PVC pipe that fits together, and paint brushes.
- Dressing Room Station with a vanity or table and bench stocked with costume jewelry, a hall tree with hats, jackets, feather boas, and scarves.
- Laundry Station with various sets of colorful socks, towels, a laundry basket, and an ironing board.

It is necessary to have all staff, leadership, and family members trained in a dementia-aware care approach in order to use these life stations effectively. The idea that simply setting these life stations up and then expecting the residents to use them on their own is not what happens! The most successful and engaging activity outcomes will emerge when everyone connects and takes positive action together with the dementia-challenged adult. I travel all over the country consulting in hundreds of beautifully set up memory care communities, complete with meticulously designed life stations. However, if there is not a program that sufficiently trains and raises dementia-awareness and practices this very different care approach for all, these life stations often sit unused and gather dust.

Helping the resident take part in life station activities can play a significant part in dealing with challenging behaviors. Knowing what helps to calm or divert a person when they are restless or distressed is very important. And a team approach to engagement is best to support all activities, for example, when the care staff sees an individual exhibiting distracting behavior in the ongoing scheduled group activity, they can step in and utilize the dementia-aware approach of guiding this individual to a life station, creating a personal meaningful moment with the one who is unable to successfully engage with the group at that time. Importantly, don't give up. Mistakes and failures will happen but don't let the person with dementia feel like a failure. Keep trying, remain creative, and don't be afraid to try a different approach. If the approach is successful—repeat, repeat, repeat. If it is not successful, back up and change the approach, the environment, and the activity.

I often have the opportunity to observe similar challenges firsthand that so many family members, professional caregivers, activity leaders, and social engagement directors struggle with as they attempt to engage and connect with their loved one, clients, or residents who are experiencing advancing dementia symptoms. Based on what I have observed and learned over the years, most professional and family dementia caregivers continually seek to find ways to successfully engage individuals, as well as those in a group setting, in meaningful, yet "dementia-appropriate" activities. There is a constant search to get past this unending struggle to connect, stay connected, and then manage to keep each individual, as well as every member within a group, mentally active and physically engaged. And, to make it even more challenging, there may be success in a group setting with a few individuals and complete nonengagement with others. How do you join together and maintain a level of enjoyment and participation with everyone? Why is finding appropriate activities such a challenge in dementia care?

When you were a baby, you didn't know how to walk, talk, play, eat, or go to the toilet. You had to learn to process or think about how to do all of these things. As you grow, you keep learning new things every day. All this learning and processing is stored in your brain. Your brain also helps you to put together all the steps you learned in the right order so you continue to succeed in processing all of the steps in the correct sequence.

A healthy brain is so good at accessing this information, thinking, and solving problems that you don't even notice it working. Tasks that you've practiced many times start to seem simple; but even simple tasks use many different parts of our brain in amazingly complex ways. Think about all the different steps and processes involved in getting yourself a glass of water or driving a car.

When a person has a loss of brain function from a cause of dementia symptoms, their brain starts to struggle with the necessary processing steps our healthy brain accesses without having to stop and think about how to do this, taking for granted how much thinking or processing this actually takes. Individuals with dementia symptoms begin to struggle with accessing all of the things they have learned or have difficulty putting them in the right order. At first, dementia-challenged adults might struggle with accessing and thinking of words or associating a face with a name. They might not be able to process that they just told a story a few minutes ago and tell the story again. Their brain might not be able to access the information of where they put something or get confused when they're trying to do the things they have done on autopilot for years. As the cause of the dementia further affects more of their brain, a person with dementia symptoms starts to lose the ability to reason and understand more involved intellectual undertakings. They might not recognize what objects are or what they're used for. They might have trouble with one or more of the steps needed to complete a task. They might get halfway through one thing and start something else instead. Things that used to be easy become very difficult.

Over time, everything they have learned since they were babies might disappear from their brain. They may find it really difficult to process tasks (activities of daily living) like getting dressed, washing, eating, or going to the toilet. They might not know where they are and get lost easily. They may have trouble keeping themselves safe. Often this culminates in people with dementia symptoms losing interest in activities they used to enjoy and being less likely to take part or even try them. And their ability to learn new activities can be lost as well.

They will need even more help and support from other people. They need those caring for them to step up and proactively "think for them," including helping them to engage and participate in meaningful social activities.

Perceptions and Approaches

A person with dementia still needs good quality of life, but without some assistance from families and caregivers, it is much more difficult for them to achieve purpose and pleasure. There are many ways to plan, come up with ideas, and provide appropriate activities for people experiencing loss and dementia symptoms, and these ideas, perceptions, and approaches can be adapted and used effectively in the home for an individual as well as for many within the long-term care setting.

Ideally, activities should

- compensate for lost abilities, whether physical, emotional, and/or social;
- promote self-esteem and provide feelings of accomplishment and value;
- maintain residual skills and not involve new learning;
- provide an opportunity for enjoyment, pleasure, and social contact; and
- be sensitive to the person's cultural background.

Dementia-challenged adults often have difficulty with visual perception and coordination.

- Ensure that surfaces are uncluttered, with few distractions and as little noise as possible.
- Maintain good lighting (without glare).
- Establish easy in-and-out seating and correct work heights.
- Use plastic containers to help avoid breakages.

Don't choose activities that reinforce inadequacy or increase stress. Levels of ability can change from day to day. Activities can be put aside and tried another time if they were not successful or enjoyable in the moment. To achieve the most success when carrying out activities, consider the time of the day when the person is at their best. For example, sometimes walking is best done in the morning or the early afternoon. For people who become restless later in the day or who have had a particularly long or meaningless day, a late afternoon walk may be better.

Understanding the person as an individual with dementia symptoms will help you to plan appropriate activities for them. This means knowing the person's former lifestyle, work history, hobbies, recreational and social interests, past travel experience, and significant life events. Make use of skills that have not been forgotten, such as buttering bread, washing up, or watering, sweeping, and raking in the garden. These are also ways in which the person with dementia can contribute to the household or community and feel useful. Encourage them to have something that is their responsibility, no matter how small.

As dementia causes the more recent memories to disappear, many memories from the past begin to feel more and more like now. When you are carrying out any other difficult care task or activity of daily living with the person who has dementia, frame your approach in a way that is familiar to the person. Doing so will help you enhance communication with the past feelings and memories where the person now resides. By using common memorabilia or topics from the past in your conversations, you can build the necessary trust. In a world of handheld electronic devices, instant communication, and fast food, we do not think in terms of the technologies that were used in the early twentieth century. Many of these gadgets have become impractical, but what is obsolete to us in a practical sense could be a gold mine for fostering great conversations with the person who has dementia, forming bonds as we enter into that person's world of fond memories.

Items of nostalgia can be used to redirect your loved one or client to a sense of familiarity and security, especially if they have a special meaning to the person you are caring for. For example, a person who worked for a long time as a secretary would relate to a manual typewriter. Someone who enjoyed church music might like to talk about the old pump-style church organ or a homemaker, about the wringer-style washer or party-line telephone. Discussing these items can help you develop a social history that is customized to the person's past individual experience. Here is a list of such items to consider talking about when working with your loved one or client. You may be able to show the person some of these items or give them to him to handle (or keep!):

- party lines on the telephone, along with a crank or rotary-dial telephone or a telephone operator who heard all the community's gossip
- pump-style organs to accompany the church choir
- wringer washing machines and washboards
- coal heaters or stoves, with the familiar coal bin and coal chute to the basement
- toilets that flushed with a chain
- pedal-driven sewing machines
- manual typewriters
- cars that started with a crank in the front
- glass milk bottles delivered to the door by a horse-drawn cart or truck
- the Good Humor ice cream man
- doctors who made house calls
- glass Coca-Cola bottles in a wooden carrier
- bottle caps lined with cork
- the malt shop on the corner
- a juke box
- penny candy
- S&H green stamps—filling the books and buying items at the stamp store
- sock hops, poodle skirts, and the jitterbug
- the Charleston and flappers
- the Iron Curtain and fallout shelters
- live radio shows, such as *Walter Winchell, Jack Benny, The Bickersons,* or *The Shadow*—with one sponsor and its famous slogan "You can trust your car to the man who wears the star."

- favorite vintage TV game shows:
  - *Beat the Clock*
  - *Concentration*
  - *I've Got a Secret*
  - *Truth or Consequences*
  - *What's My Line?*
  - *You Bet Your Life* (a.k.a. *The Groucho Show*)

Take the time to talk about these and other long-ago memories. The person you are caring for was probably greatly influenced by at least one if not many of the subjects on this list. The more you discover about your loved one or client's past, the more easily you will be able to reach her through her unique dementia dialect.

Try not to overstimulate the person with dementia symptoms. Be selective with outings. Avoid crowds, constant movement, and noise, which many people with dementia symptoms find overwhelming. Simple and unhurried activities are best. Give the time and space necessary to allow the person to do as much as possible. Focus on one thing at a time. Communicate one instruction at a time. Break down activities into simple, manageable steps. A person with dementia symptoms may enjoy an outing, even if they do not remember where they have been. What is important is that the moment is enjoyed, and in the moment, they experience feelings of love, safety, security, and value.

It can be helpful to write out a customized activities care plan working with all of those involved in their care, including family members, clergy, professional care providers, neighbors, and friends. This will help make sure that the activities are consistent and are suited to the individual needs of the person with dementia symptoms.

For many people with dementia, a sense of movement and rhythm is often retained. Listening to music, dancing, or having contact with babies, children, or animals provides positive feelings. People with dementia often have excellent memories of past events and looking through old photos, memorabilia, and books can help the person to recall and enjoy earlier times. The opportunity to relive treasured moments can be deeply satisfying. If reading skills have deteriorated, make recordings for them. Locate picture books and magazines in the person's areas of interest.

Some sensory experiences that the person with dementia might like include

- enjoying a hand, neck, or foot massage
- brushing their hair
- smelling fresh flowers
- using essential oils and fragrances
- stroking an animal or differently textured fabrics
- visiting an herb farm or a flower show
- looking through a box containing things that the person has found interesting in the past, such as costume jewelry, postcards, or greeting cards

Keeping individuals with dementia symptoms actively engaged in everyday activities and cognitively challenging tasks is beneficial for both body and mind and, in some cases, it can even slow the progression of the disease. Staying active and engaged can help to reduce dementia sleep problems as well. Keep the person involved. Activities don't only pass the time but also help the person retain important skills and provide enjoyment and social contact. Don't feel you have to fill every minute of the day! Quiet times are important too—including sleep.

Lose your preconceived notions of how the activity should be done or what the outcome is supposed to be, as those with varying levels of loss and different dementia symptoms may not be capable of understanding the goal of an activity. Just enjoy the process and the current moment of doing, it is so comforting when you are just present with them. When we think of "activities" for people living with any cause of dementia symptoms, we need to broaden the scope of that word. In fact, as the disease progresses and the person is able to do less, what is considered "activities" for the person should broaden more. It can be easy to assume that when a person is no longer communicating with words or is spending much of their day in bed, the emphasis will be on keeping the person physically comfortable and activities become less relevant. However, a person in the advanced stages of dementia can still experience emotions such as loneliness, boredom, or frustration.

A person might no longer be able to move independently or hold a conversation. However, many people with dementia will respond positively to close one-to-one attention using the eyes to communicate or hands to touch and make a connection. Many people with dementia will sense when we are not fully present and are less likely to connect with us in any meaningful way if this is the case. If we are not paying full attention, we might also miss simple movements or sounds from the person attempting to communicate something.

Don't forget to look after yourself as a family caregiver, just as we all need to consider ways to support staff in the professional setting too. Spending time with people in the advanced stages of dementia is personally challenging and everyone needs support. Dementia care leadership needs to give time to their teams to discuss difficult encounters but most importantly to praise the effort and encourage the staff member to try again in a different moment, as the person with dementia might respond very differently.

CHAPTER FIFTEEN

Susan

Dealing with Disruption

With Alicia Murray

Susan had finally accepted the promotion she had worked so hard for over her entire career. She had been offered the job numerous times in the past, but she had turned it down because her children were still little and the position demanded longer hours.

But now she was up for it! And she was finally the manager of her own department at the age of 42. She felt this was a new chapter in her life, and she was enjoying the rewards of her expertise and dedication.

Then, one day, her cell phone rang. Her heart dropped as she heard the voice of her sister, who rarely called unless there was an emergency. Perhaps her sister was calling to congratulate her on the promotion: "Hey, Sis, what's going on?"

"Susan, you need to get down to the hospital right away. I think Mom may have had a stroke!" Their mother, confused and agitated, had been found wandering down the middle of the street. Her speech had been slurred, and she had been walking with an unsteady gait. Not knowing what to do when she got the call from a neighbor, Susan's sister had dropped everything and rushed her mother to the hospital.

The next four hours in the hospital were agonizing, as Susan and her sister tried to get information from the doctors. It felt like they were in the ultimate boxing championship and were losing badly. Then they finally got the answers.

Susan's mother had had a series of small strokes, and her sudden change in behavior was caused by vascular dementia. The doctor suggested she stay overnight for monitoring and also recommended placing her in a rehabilitation center or taking her home and getting professional caregivers to assist her. The doctor told both daughters that the mother they had known and loved was still in there but was now presented in a different package. She would probably not remember a lot of things, and she would also need twenty-four-hour care because her strokes had affected her memory and judgment and left a portion of her left side paralyzed.

Susan and her sister went to a nearby diner to talk over what needed to be done for their mother. Since their father had died a few years earlier, their mother had lived on her own, not wanting to go into one of those "old folks' homes."

To complicate matters, Susan's sister, who was quite a few years younger, had just gotten married and was planning on moving out of state the following month. Her husband had been offered a new position with his company, and she had been transferred within hers. They had already sold their home and were living in temporary housing until all the paperwork for his job came through. She offered to help pay for a caregiver for their mother but thought it would be more economical if their mother moved in with Susan rather than going to a care facility. Susan agreed that she could save money by hiring a professional caregiver during the day but taking care of their mother herself at night. The sale of their mother's home would help raise money for the caregivers.

That night, Susan called to get pricing for many different in-home care companies. Making the calculations, she figured that if the caregiver was there for six hours a day, she and her older kids could manage the rest. So she made arrangements for an in-home caregiver to work at her house five days a week for one month.

That month was far more difficult than anyone could have imagined. Susan constantly got phone calls at work from her mother. Her mother said that she did not need a caregiver and insisted that she could move back to her own house. The phone calls, with the same conversation, kept coming every couple of hours. Her mother would tell the caregiver that she was going to lie down for a nap, and then she would sneak off to call Susan, over and over again.

Susan knew she could not keep this up. Her boss had already talked to her about the excessive personal phone calls and the amount of time she had taken for doctors' appointments, suggesting she take some time off to figure out another solution. Susan had many projects due on a deadline, and she worried that a temporary leave of absence would jeopardize her career. But she could not stop the phone calls and she could not rearrange the doctors' appointments for after work.

What was she going to do? Not only were her newfound opportunities slipping away, she was also physically exhausted. Plus, the family was in an uproar over the disruptions that the changes had caused. And if she lost her job, the financial implications would spell disaster.

Lessons Learned

Susan is one of many caregivers trying to juggle the daily responsibilities of work and caregiving. Attorney Todd C. Ratner, who specializes in elder law and estate planning, notes that sixteen million Americans find themselves sandwiched between two generations, struggling to raise kids while caring for an aging parent and holding down a full-time job. This multidirectional tug-of-war can be the leading cause of stress in family caregiving. Overwhelmed and unable to meet the constant demands, many caregivers tell us, "There's just not enough time in the day!" And it is so difficult to ask for help.

Well, I cannot make the days longer, but I can help make the days easier. When I started working with Susan, she was very upset and frustrated with her mother's challenging behaviors—not only the phone calls that would not stop, but also the late-night wandering and the same questions repeated endlessly. Susan, her family, and her job were all suffering.

I asked Susan to buy a tape recorder and record short messages that the professional caregiver could play for her mother throughout the day. The caregiver would introduce the recordings by telling Susan's mother that Susan had left a message on the answering machine: "Hi,

Mom! I wanted to let you know that I'm in meetings all day, but I'm thinking of you and will call back later."

This little trick stopped the excessive daily phone calls. Every few days, Susan would re-record the messages and add different stories that her mother could reminisce about. It relieved some of her mother's stress and allowed Susan to focus on her job. Susan also started having the daytime caregiver take her mother to her doctors' appointments. Susan would follow up with the doctor by telephone to discuss her mother's health. Now she could get a full day's work done.

She also enrolled her mother in an adult daycare program through the local hospital, giving her three days a week out of the house. Susan realized that she needed to access as many of the senior community resources as possible. Asking for assistance from friends, family, neighbors, professionals, and the community did not make her a failure after all!

Susan joined a caregiver support group that met in the evening one day a month. By sharing her struggles with others who had similar challenges, she learned that she was not alone. Every three months, Susan's entire family, including her children, were invited to a meeting devoted to family matters. These meetings were designed to develop a team spirit, empowering everyone as they discussed the difficulties that filtered down to even the youngest child. They also promoted proactive approaches to caregiving. The family gained a clearer understanding of dementia and learned tips for sharing more meaningful moments with Susan's mother.

Above all, Susan realized that she had to take care of herself, or she would eventually burn out. She focused on eating right, exercising, and squeezing in extra time for activities she enjoyed, like taking a hot bath and reading her favorite novels. Getting restful sleep became a high priority. She made sure to thank all of her supportive coworkers. A few of them had their own heavy family responsibilities, and they agreed to ease the burdens by helping out with each other's projects.

After six months, Susan's mother developed some serious health problems and had to be placed in a skilled nursing facility that could provide her the medical care she needed. The family knew they had pursued every resource to help keep her at home as long as possible.

Perceptions and Approaches

Many of the caregivers who attend my presentations share their own stories and experiences. A common theme among them is the tension that caregiving puts on their entire families, not just on the person who is the primary caregiver. Caring for a person with dementia can put a strain on even the most well-balanced family.

There are disruptions in schedules, meals, family events, and personal space. The family's finances can also be adversely affected—even drained—not only because the family is paying for private professional care, but often also because family caregivers must change jobs or take on additional jobs to work around their new roles. Because the person with dementia requires so much care, young children and teenagers often don't get the time and attention they need, and this disruption may happen just as the children need more of their parents' time, for one reason or another. The emotional toll on everyone can be extreme. Before taking on the daunting challenge of caring for a relative with dementia in the home, family members must anticipate what this will mean in terms of the day-to-day dynamic and factor that into the decision.

To cope with the challenge, you must access all of your options for support, including local community resources. Never be afraid to ask for help. Asking for help is a necessary part of your caregiving role. If you are able to maintain an open-minded approach to problem-solving, you will feel more effective and you will be less stressed.

CHAPTER SIXTEEN

Grace

Moving beyond Guilt

With Alicia Murray

Grace was a very active woman. She loved to go to church, take pottery classes at the local community center, and spend time with her husband, Ned. He was her confidante, her soul mate. When Ned was diagnosed with Alzheimer's, there was no option in her mind other than to become his devoted full-time caregiver.

Ned's diagnosis was heart-wrenching. Grace talked about the emotions that crashed around her: the grief of knowing there was no cure, the loneliness of missing her partner and friend, and the anxiety of knowing he would not be with her much longer. Taking care of her husband now took her entire day. She no longer attended her pottery class or went to church. She felt that she had to be there with Ned every minute.

Grace was exhausted. Further, she had completely isolated herself from the outside world. Family members offered to help her, but she always turned them down. Like so many other caregivers, she felt guilty asking someone else for assistance to do something that she truly believed she ought to be able to do herself.

With Alzheimer disease, memory loss and challenging behaviors become more noticeable as the disease progresses. Grace was working harder and harder to redirect Ned's activities. Getting him to do simple things—things that in the beginning stages of the disease he had been able to do with just a little help from her—now required a lot more effort. Grace also began to have her own health issues.

The family had to intervene, and they called me for help. As Grace and I talked about her situation, she realized that she was on a destructive path and that she needed to make changes to preserve her own health. She made a list of all the family members who had offered to help, and she called them to set up a schedule when they would come and sit with her husband. Grace began attending church on a regular basis again, and she signed up to take her favorite pottery class.

She also joined an Alzheimer's support group, where she could talk with family caregivers who were in the same situation she was in. Grace found the support group to be very helpful. Because there were family caregivers whose loved ones were in different stages of dementia, she learned from some of them and taught others what she had learned from her own experience.

The caregiving journey is full of lessons. For Grace, giving the gift of experience to other caregivers was the ticket to relieving her feelings of guilt and working through the new and sometimes difficult emotions she struggled with. Best of all, once she was relieved of guilt, she was able to share many more meaningful moments with her husband.

Lessons Learned

Grace's story brings us to an extremely common caregiving emotion: guilt. Guilt is remorse for having done something wrong. But would it have been wrong for Grace to ask for help in addressing her own needs? Did Grace have to feel guilty about taking one hour a day for herself? Should she feel guilty about needing a break from her caregiving duties? The answer is obvious: *no.*

Grace was a wonderful wife who had taken on the caregiving role and had not thought twice about her own needs. But guilt keeps family members from doing things for themselves, and not doing anything for themselves leads to physical, mental, and emotional stress—and, possibly, breakdowns. Many family caregivers feel guilty as a result of being faced with one of the hardest jobs they will ever do.

They feel guilty if they have fun. They feel guilty if they leave their loved one home alone or with someone else. They feel guilty that they cannot do it all. Guilt sneaks in on these family caregivers regardless of how effective they are or how much time they spend doing this job. This guilt becomes a thunderhead on a sunny day, clouding one's judgment and cultivating sadness and even depression.

Perceptions and Approaches

Unjustified guilt is destructive in many ways. Perhaps its worst aspect is that it makes you as a caregiver believe you are a failure, when in reality, caregivers are the heroes and leaders in the face of dementia. To help you cope with the guilt and any other strong emotions you are experiencing you must first understand this concept. Then you need to find out what's causing your feelings of guilt, talk about your feelings, and take time for yourself.

Caregivers heap undue pressure on themselves and feel guilty about things they do not need to feel guilty about. Moving past guilt can be hard, but you owe it to yourself to find freedom from it. As Dorothy Womack wrote, "Release the guilt you carry and listen with your heart—you will truly find [that] your loved ones not only dwell in peace, but wish the same for you as well."

CHAPTER SEVENTEEN

Virginia

Laughter Is Therapeutic

With Alicia Murray

Virginia was a full-time caregiver for her mother who had dementia. One morning, Virginia was cooking breakfast when her mother came into the kitchen complaining that her pants were too tight. Virginia turned around from the stove to see what her mother was talking about and nearly burst into laughter. Her mother was standing there with her legs through the sleeves of her blouse, trying to pull them up past her knees.

Holding it all in, Virginia gave her mother an *affirmative response* without making her feel silly or stupid for trying to put on a blouse the same way she would put on a pair of pants. She guided her mother back to her room, taking full responsibility for the shrinking pants by explaining she must have washed them in hot water and shrunk them accidentally. She helped her mother get dressed and then assisted her to the table. While her mother was eating breakfast, Virginia sneaked into the bathroom and laughed so hard she had tears rolling down her face.

Lessons Learned

Sometimes it can feel like there's not a lot in your life to laugh about. But laughter is a wonderful stress buster and has great effects on your body. In fact, it increases blood flow, decreases stress hormones, boosts metabolism, and helps put our problems into perspective. Most importantly, it can help us keep our sanity in overwhelming situations.

I recently met an amazing woman, Dani Klein Modisett, who not only learned about the positive power of laughter shortly after her mother was diagnosed with Alzheimer's; she then courageously took this powerful dementia-awareness of the importance of laughing together and shares it with everyone in such a unique and valuable way. Here is her story:

I love what Laura says here about giving you "permission to laugh." Seven years ago, my mother was diagnosed with Alzheimer's. After moving her from New York City to Los Angeles to be near me and my family, I found that she was becoming depressed. A comic myself, I thought surely there must be a way to make my mother laugh. As her daughter, with a lifetime of history together, I was not the woman for the job. I thought, maybe I should hire a professional! So I did. A friend of mine in New York City knew a woman in Los Angeles who was a comic and wanted to work with seniors. She came and met my mother. She got down at her eye level and talked honestly to her. "You probably don't want to talk to me, you're probably thinking who is this schmuck talking to me right now?!" My mother heard this familiar Yiddish word and her eyes lit up and she started laughing. The comic repeated it and she laughed more. It was contagious, as all laughter is, and we all started laughing. I hired the woman on the spot. She visited with my mother about eight hours a week and within just a few visits, my mother felt better. She started eating again and engaging with her community. I knew immediately the importance of these exchanges. They were honest and joyful and fully engaged. Other people started asking for a comedian to work with their loved one, and I did the same for them. Honestly, I had no intention of working in the field of dementia care, but the results these "comedy care" sessions were achieving, in terms of engagement and real laughter, were undeniable.

A year ago, I launched a company called "Laughter On Call," in addition to bringing comedians to work one on one with your loved ones; I also teach workshops to caregivers and family members in how to create more laughter under these toughest of circumstances. Drawing on the curriculum I used teaching stand up at [the] University of California at Los Angeles, I picked out the most relevant tools that comedians use to create connection with people. In that first interaction between the comedian and my mother, we already saw the power of honesty, of not pretending something isn't happening when it is, and how equally important it is to let go of any negative moments quickly, to accept an imperfect moment, to release any idea of a perfect visit or conversation and allow yourselves to be fully present to the moment you are having. Another great tool is to take time to appreciate even the smallest detail, the softness of a fabric, someone's beautiful smile, the smell of freshly baked anything, and most importantly to not be afraid to be silly! My mother no longer has much language, a word or two now and then, but she absolutely responds to my face and my tone of voice and dancing. Being silly for or with your loved one is very freeing and brings a completely different energy to rooms that are often mired in sadness.

Of course, we must not forget the key point that Laura hits very strongly, don't argue with a person in the struggle of experiencing loss of brain function and dementia symptoms. Saying "yes and," is one of the essential tenets of improvisational comedy and it turns out there is no better place to make use of this comedy tool than when you are dealing with a loved one or client with any cause of dementia symptoms. Rather than shutting down their belief we will be much more successful in engaging if we join them in their feelings and use creative interventions, such as agreeing that they are indeed in Coney Island and need to get to the bus before dark! You will experience more successful engagement as you go along with them and utilize positive action statements about the place and what the bus is like and where it's going and suggest maybe having a snack before you leave. It is a great opportunity to let your imagination run, too. In doing this, you get ahead of any possible tension, resistance or negativity in your interactions. As the kids say, it's all good. Isolation and fear are such a big part of the dementia experience and the greatest gift you can give your loved one, client or patient is to comfort them by smiling and saying yes whenever possible. And hopefully you get the chance to hold their hands and dance with them too.

I am giving this book to everyone I know, including a close family member, because they have an in-law that was just diagnosed with Alzheimer's!

Dani Klein Modisett, Founder and CEO of Laughter On Call

Perceptions and Approaches

Think about what you can do to bring laughter into your life. I enjoy spending time with my family and friends. The young children in my family are full of laughter and hearing their pure joy never fails to bring a smile to my face.

Even watching a funny show or movie with your loved one or client can be therapeutic. One woman told us a story about the time she spent caring for her mother. Her mother's favorite show while growing up was *I Love Lucy*, so the daughter bought the entire collection. They would spend a couple of hours a day laughing together, and she explained that those moments would forever stay within her heart.

Translation: Start laughing now! I hear many caregivers say, "I'm sure I'll be able to laugh about this someday." The sooner you quit waiting for "someday," the more you will enjoy your caregiving role today.

Sometimes people with dementia say and do things that are funny, like Virginia's mother's shrinking "pants." *Give yourself permission to laugh today.* Find humor in a difficult situation, if you can. Your caregiving role may be hard, but each day is precious, so take time to enjoy the moments that you share. As comedian Bob Newhart reportedly said, "Laughter gives us distance. It allows us to step back from an event, deal with it, and then move on."

CHAPTER EIGHTEEN

Maria and Andreas

In Sickness and in Health

Maria and Andreas's marriage was not perfect, but it was based in good, solid love. Andreas had a vivacious personality and was well-regarded and active in the local Greek and church communities. After thirty years of star work performance in his long-standing job in health-care IT management, Andreas received a lower performance review from an unhappy (obviously who was not dementia-aware) manager and was blamed for serious communication problems at his job. These problems, unfortunately, were due to early signs, symptoms, and behaviors of a then unrecognized but later confirmed diagnosis of fron-totemporal degeneration (FTD)—of which there are two types, a behavioral variant and primary progressive aphasia. There were many other early signs of his loss of brain function and subsequent dementia symptoms showing up in his marriage and home life. At the time, Maria was unaware that these changes were a part of his inability to process the information he had so easily processed in the past, before the FTD damage, about his relationships at home and outside the home. He became uncharacteristically verbally and physically aggressive, presented narcissistic and frightening abusive behavior, such as threatening nonstop and in front of their kids to kick Maria out of the house if she didn't return to the bedroom to sleep. Maria felt so threatened by these out of character changes in his behavior toward her that she left the home, served papers, and they headed into divorce. This was the beginning of their bewildering dementia journey, although at the time no one was aware of what was happening and where this change of condition was going to take them. Because there was no local family nearby on either side to provide either emotional or physical support, Maria was suddenly thrust into the role of a single mother, sole provider and, unbeknownst to her at the time, soon to be a full-time caregiver for a loved one with FTD dementia.

After Maria's eighteen months of separation and nearing the finish line of a completed divorce, her daughter alerted Maria to the fact that the mortgage on the house where Andreas was still residing wasn't being paid. This was the "straw that broke the camel's back." Maria recognized that something was very wrong with Andreas's health, as this was the complete opposite of who he was and how he had always conducted his financial life. Maria became convinced that she had to step back, pause the legal action of divorce, and take immediate action to support her obviously ill husband and the father of their children.

Throughout the time of being back in his life, Maria found herself having to spend immense amounts of time advocating medically to get an expedited diagnosis, apply for support from social security, put out many financial fires, and repair effects of home and relationship neglect. She experienced great emotional benefit from planning, expediting, and helping him return to his home country for a family visit and, on a regular basis, arranging and together taking part in appropriate activities and outings with their children. Anosognosia (a far-reaching lack of awareness of impairment, often a dementia symptom; see chapter 4) was one of the many hard challenges and yet at times a big blessing. If Andreas had been aware of his loss, it would have probably made it a lot worse. Rather, they utilized successful creative interventions and dementia-aware communication strategies, at times simply because he could not understand that he had any serious loss that was affecting major cognitive functions, including his ability to process and reason. Gradually the children and Maria witnessed Andreas present more consistent calmness and loving behaviors, and all enjoyed more meaningful moments with fewer of his challenging dementia behaviors interfering on this often roller-coaster-like dementia journey. Through prayer, courage, and empowerment from dementia-aware education and coaching, the kids and Maria decided to move back in. While entering the unknown dementia world was a gamble, they unanimously felt they understood the basics and had a firm foundation of awareness that would provide the skills and support necessary to safely join him as a family on this wild and crazy dementia journey.

Maria's most basic feelings of love for him were, over time, revitalized and continued to grow. The three of them were thrilled that the family was back together, yet conscious of their newfound dementia-awareness, they realized they were not stopping, fixing, or changing the decline, and only successfully managing it. They continued to stay sensitive and observant to any progressive changes and remained vigilant to what modifications lay ahead. They all agreed that the dementia-awareness, deeper understanding, and transformed perception of dementia, along with the affirming strategies and upgraded skills, brought them together and better prepared them for the dementia care marathon they now took part in day to day.

Lessons Learned

Dementia caregiving is all about managing loss and change. It is about learning to simultaneously witness and then grieve the daily losses while, at the same time, developing new skills to handle the constant changes. There can be discomfort being on the early end of a learning curve of new skills, and trying out new ways to manage behavior at the same time that you're grieving is something no one ever expects to have to do at all, let alone for an extended period of months or even years. It is about learning how to make everything into your "new normal" as opposed to stressing on how to attempt to do the impossible by reverting back to the "old normal." It is about recognizing and accepting loss of brain function and the presentation of dementia symptoms as early as possible and not ignoring or staying in the short-term security of dementia-denial.

Instead it is about becoming proactively dementia-aware, looking deep into progressive loss and changes over time, and being aware of the fact that dementia is not all about the changes that occur with

memory loss. Your spouse may have difficulty remembering information even if it is recently learned, however, presenting some decline in
memory may just be the "tip of the iceberg." Is your spouse suddenly
and uncharacteristically acting paranoid, such as accusing you of having an affair when it is not true? Are they unusually irritable, angry,
aggressive, argumentative, verbally or physically abusive? Are they getting lost while driving or walking? Do they have trouble finding words
in the middle of a sentence? Are they repeating questions soon after
you have given the answer?

When dementia happens to a marriage it is about losing what may
have been a long-standing partnership and lifelong friendship that is
now developing into more of a parent-child relationship. It becomes
necessary to admit that these personality and behavior changes will
make the prior couple relationship end.

So how does the healthy spouse learn to cope?

- Keep in the forefront of your mind that you cannot stop, fix, or
  change the cause, the decline, or the challenges; you can only
  manage them.
- Remain calm, confident, patient, and present with them in the
  moment—in the same way you would not get angry or frustrated with someone with high blood pressure or diabetes.
- Line up support such as nonprofit crisis therapy, dementia-
  specific support groups for yourself and all family members.
- Pursue ongoing dementia-aware education and coaching (reading this book as well as seeking out personal consultations
  with Ms. Wayman or other dementia-aware professionals
  and resources) will be lifesavers.
- Practice appreciating and cultivating your spouse's current
  capabilities, what they can still do today. Work on stopping
  yourself from getting emotionally stuck or dwell in lost
  capabilities—as sad as they are to witness.
- Accept that there may be a time when the care needs are beyond
  your abilities or resources. As much as you know you can't
  stop the feelings of guilt later on for tough decisions, it will
  be necessary to make them (such as having to place your

spouse into a care community). Know you can live in a way that has a good chance of bringing a sense of pride and peace when you look back and recognize you did the best you could and made all care decisions with the best of intentions and with the most educated awareness that ensured your loved one always received appropriate levels of care.

- Build your caregiving village. Ask for support from family, friends, neighbors, professionals, and your medical community.

When dementia symptoms happen to a marriage, there is significant emotional loss for the healthy spouse as well. Here are some ways to approach these emotional losses, supporting you as the caregiver, inside this mystifying dementia journey:

- Accept that your marriage is permanently changed and will continue to change.
- Continue to educate yourself (become dementia-aware).
- Understand your spouse's changes in behavior are not intentional.
- Know that feelings of hopelessness and resentment are common.
- Understand that intimacy may change.
- Start a "feelings" journal where you can jot down how all of this "feels."
- Find a support group; being around others who make you feel safe enough to share your honest thoughts and feelings can be so freeing.
- Focus on the positives.

Maria and the children are driven to do all they can now. One of the most important things Maria felt she did was to structure their lives so she and the children can enjoy Andreas in the moment. For example, she managed to reduce her work hours and schedule more family and vacation time. Friends have disappeared. Family doesn't understand or agree. Caregivers, volunteers, and reunited neighbors are their new family friends.

Ongoing positive interactions with Andreas in a manner that helps him feel love, comfort, safety, and value still arise and remain relatively easy for them. Establishing a daily routine that accomplishes these goals is the main reason for this success. The overwhelming household, financial, and firefighting tasks trickled down to a minimum over time, allowing more time for Maria to focus on the increased caregiving demands that kicked in later. One of the many challenges facing them now is establishing boundaries for each one of them amid his increasing care needs so that they don't lose who they are, end up with a broken spirit, or stop living their lives.

Perceptions and Approaches

Andreas continued to decline and, within one year of his initial diagnosis, his SLUMS score (Saint Louis University Mental Status Examination, or SLUMS, is a method of screening for Alzheimer's and other kinds of dementia) showed a devastating reduction from eleven to four. He is now unable to drive, understand basic concepts or multiple-step instructions, and continues to present many more devastating symptoms and loss. Yet Maria and the kids are determined to keep him home as long as possible. The three of them know as he slips away, they need to get stronger. They work on putting each other first, so that they can grow in mental, spiritual, and physical health. The daily events can draw them into crisis reaction, so they practice making conscious choices every day to live their lives in line with everyone's best interests and values as much as possible. They don't want to just survive this; they plan to come out better on the other side and thrive.

As Andreas entered later stages, the journey became more of a spiritual experience. Being present moment by moment, enjoying each other, being grateful for these moments and the sacrifice of things that were once important has redefined and raised the bar of love and deepened the entire family's life experience beyond their imagination. Dementia-aware coaching has been the handholding necessary and a big part of why Maria does not feel alone like so many of her peer FTD dementia spouse/caregivers express.

Maria recently shared with me her mission statement as a wife/caregiver:

- To remain courageous, vulnerable, and authentic
- To continue to "openly share her heart, seeking first to understand, then to be understood," (from the book, *The 7 Habits of Highly Effective People* by Steven R. Covey)
- To seek wisdom, follow her intuition and conscience, and maintain presence in the moment

Maria's previous special education training combined with her newly acquired dementia-awareness has taught her to be conscious of her response to her husband's increasingly more limited mental energy and slower response time. She is aware that she has a choice in how to use her own mental energy during these moments. She works hard to be selective in the moment about the use of her time. Maria also shared with me that she is working on an in-the-moment routine that helps her stay focused on her own intentions for when she is alone or next to her husband. She wants to be connected to his feelings in a way which makes him feel completely understood and that his thoughts are important to her, even when he doesn't have the words or congruent actions to send the message accurately.

She runs through this checklist to help her manage her own feelings in the moment:

- What do I do with the extra mental energy that the moment requires of just being by his side?
- Do I feel sad?
- Do I judge what he says or does?
- Do I attempt to understand his intention?
- Am I impatient?
- Am I too busy with my to-do list thoughts?
- Do I practice deep breathing?

Because this is so difficult to achieve, she feels she is a work-in-progress, reminding herself that this is a spiritual journey of deep connection that takes such commitment and requires constant attention that she needs to do a better job of taking care of herself, so she is better able to accomplish this effectively. Trying to shift judgment of herself from "this is too hard, I'm too tired, I can't do this" to "this is a lifetime of skills and awareness that is acquired and perfected over time and requires lots of practice." Maria admits she is not there yet, a simple thought that shows respect to herself. She is not there *yet*. She understands she needs to be as kind to herself as she is to Andreas and replace judgment with recognition and appreciation for all that she is doing now. She does not keep a journal or do anything reflective in addition to her support groups and therapy. She feels it is necessary to spend time away from it all for respite and to reset and return rejuvenated. Maybe someday she will find solace in a journal and write, but right now, managing the daily demands and enjoying one another has all of her attention.

Maria, although she recognizes the horrific loss and devastating pain that comes with a cause of dementia, feels she has more opportunity in a million moments throughout the day than ever to live her personal life mission. And the impact of living this way is multiplied by Andreas's ability to feel more comfort and peace, which in turn brought a sense of comfort and peace in the home that was not experienced for many years in the past.

CHAPTER NINETEEN

Beatrice and Henry

The Power of Gratitude

Beatrice and Henry had been married for many years. After the children were grown and the house was empty, Beatrice realized she did not really have a lot in common with her husband.

She thought he could be a bit overbearing, and she did not like how he laughed at things that were not at all funny. She was extremely bothered by the way he read his newspaper in the morning at breakfast, while slurping his coffee and clanking his spoon in his cereal bowl. Just being around him made her sick. She talked with her friends about Henry and all his annoying habits and how life was not what she had imagined. She spoke of divorce, but one of her friends, who had been through a couple of nasty divorces, told her that Henry was a good man and that she should see a counselor before seeing an attorney.

Determined either to seek help or to see an attorney, she went to the counselor recommended by her friend, but not without skepticism and with anger in her heart. She asked herself, "How can this counselor help me?" As she slouched on the couch and told the counselor why she was there and the frustrating things that her lovely Henry was doing, the counselor began to smile. "Beatrice, I have an assignment for you," she said. "I want you to go home, and every day I want you to tell Henry about something that he does that you are grateful for. It has to be something new every day. It has to be honest. And it has to be done for the next two weeks. Then come back and see me again."

Needless to say, Beatrice was thoroughly upset. She had gone to the counselor to get either a solution to the situation or permission for a divorce—not to get a homework assignment. The next morning at breakfast as Henry slurped his coffee and rattled his newspaper, Beatrice rolled her eyes. "How am I going to find something about him that I am grateful for?" She stood at the counter in the kitchen staring at Henry eating his breakfast when she noticed his nails were very nicely groomed. She said to him, "Henry, I am very grateful that you always take such good care of your nails." Small but honest: she only had to think of thirteen more and she would be home free.

The next morning the gratefulness was not overflowing as she stood at the counter in the kitchen racking her brain for something she could say to Henry. Then, like a light switch being flipped on, she noticed his tie. What a nice tie that was—he always matched his ties to his suits. "Henry, you always have the best-looking ties. They always match your suits so nicely." Henry put down his newspaper, smiled, looked down at his tie and said, "This is the one you gave me for my birthday."

The next morning was a little easier. Actually, she had spent the remainder of the previous day thinking about what she would say, and before Henry could pick up his newspaper, she blurted out, "You always take such great care of your shoes. They are always so shiny and clean." Henry smiled and replied, "You look lovely today. Is that a new outfit?" Beatrice smiled and affirmed that it was.

The following days were amazing; the breakfast table had become a place where they had conversations instead of eating in silence. The compliments had become bigger and more personal. The time they spent together had become richer, and Beatrice was remembering who she had fallen in love with years ago.

When she went back to the counselor for her next appointment, the counselor was delighted with the progress Beatrice and Henry were making. The counselor explained that sometimes people take the little things in life for granted, only seeing the glass half-empty. But when you change your perspective and search for the things to be grateful for, you begin to appreciate those little things that have been overlooked.

Three months later, Beatrice and Henry were celebrating their second honeymoon.

Lessons Learned

It is hard to remember how important it is to be thankful for every-thing we have in our lives, especially when we are faced with the daunting task of caring for a loved one or client who has dementia. Research shows that caring for someone with dementia is three times harder than caring for someone with a physical ailment.

It may be difficult to find something to be grateful for, but it can be even small things like, "I'm grateful I have clean sheets or a roof over my head or shoes on my feet." In my training workshops and presen-tations, people often come up to me after class and say that they did not believe they had anything to be grateful for—but that they were surprised at the power of appreciation when they list even the little things.

Perceptions and Approaches

When working with people with dementia, look for the good in the situation. It can be the simple fact that when you visit them in their world, they are more cooperative. That is something to be thankful for, and especially if you are a caregiver who has been thrust into this position involuntarily, cooperation is a huge blessing.

By changing our perspective and focusing on the positive instead of the negative, we are able to see things more clearly and are often able to appreciate the importance of the time shared with others. We also understand just how important it is to ignore the unimportant cobwebs in the corner of the house.

If you develop the daily habit of writing at least five things you are thankful for in a gratitude journal, no matter how small they may be, you will find that it gets easier and easier to exist in a place of grate-fulness. The end result will be positively dramatic!

If you keep a journal, you can also track changes in your loved one or client, identify any potential causes of resistance or combative be-havior, and adjust your strategies accordingly. Further, if you meet with other caregivers, your journals can be excellent resources and help guide all of you as you share lessons learned.

You may feel you need the support that comes from sharing your thoughts and feelings with others. Some days you may need an empathetic ear, someone who will listen and will not judge. Other days you may need a safe place to vent. Friends and family are a great place to start.

As caregivers in our stories have discovered, a support group can give you a place to talk with other caregivers who understand the disease and know exactly what you are going through. Meeting in a group will give you an opportunity to share your own experiences, get practical suggestions that can help you, and experience the joy of helping others as well. A support group can also help you manage stress and feel less isolated.

As you proceed through your caregiving experience, recognize that you may be going through a variety of emotions, including frustration, fear, and sadness. These emotions are normal and common among caregivers, and they may come and go. Sometimes caregivers even get depressed. The person with dementia and other family members may be experiencing the same types of emotions too. If your feelings or those of your loved one are overwhelming and persistent, do not hesitate to talk to your doctor and ask for help.

Remember, you are not taking this journey alone. And keep in mind that there can be joy and fulfillment along the way.

Sean

The Puzzling Pieces of Grief

With Denise Howard

The following story is an account of how a dear, lifelong friend of mine came to devote her life to being a certified grief recovery specialist.

Sean was my firstborn child and only son. He was born when I was just 21, a child myself. As I held him and looked into his beautiful blue eyes, he brought great joy into my life, and through his birth, I saw the miracle of God for the very first time. Three and a half years later, I gave birth to Sean's little sister, Danalyn. From the moment Sean laid eyes on her, he beamed with pride. The relationship they shared was the most rewarding gift of my life, and as the years went on, they continued to grow closer and closer.

Since I was a single mom for many years, the three of us developed an extraordinary and unique bond. We spent many hours talking, laughing, playing, and growing up together. My children are my life and my heart.

On Sunday, September 19, 2004, Sean was on his way home after a late night of being out with friends. He never arrived.

On Monday morning, when I realized that Sean was not in his room sleeping, which would have been the norm, Danalyn and I knew that something was not right and we started making phone calls. Sean absolutely loved to be at home, and it was unusual for him to stay at a friend's house. Besides that, he would have contacted us.

When night came on Monday, we called the police, and the search began. For eight days, we looked, almost twenty-four hours a day, to find him. We organized search parties and had a search dog; we even had a helicopter. We made thousands of calls. It was like living in the Twilight Zone.

On the ninth day at 1:30 in the afternoon, we got the call that no parent or loved one is prepared to receive. Sean had been found dead on a heavily traveled interstate freeway near Sacramento, California. He had fallen asleep while driving and veered off the road, crashing into some trees and a sound wall. Sean had been ejected from his car and was hidden behind such dense brush that neither he nor his car could be seen from the road.

From that day on our lives were forever changed, and Danalyn and I began to understand the definition of the word "grief."

I was in shock. I was unable to think clearly or make decisions, let alone follow through with any decision I had made. I was numb and could not figure out how I was going to continue to live without dying of a broken heart. I turned to a few local churches and counselors, and while everyone wanted to console me, no one knew how to give me the help I desperately needed. Because I was unable to find any kind of support system that met my needs, I began listening, reading, and learning as much as I could about grief and how other people have survived this nightmare. Along the way, I learned many things that I now attempt to share with others when they ask for help.

I also decided to take my broken heart and reach out to other families that had lost a child. I have been doing this ever since. Focusing on others helps me to know that I am not the only one who is hurting. For those who have suffered a loss, grieving is a journey through which we will have to travel for the rest of our lives.

But there is hope. With grief professionals and friends to pray, support, and encourage each other, we can find comfort this side of heaven.

Lessons Learned

Through this tragedy, my friend, Denise Howard, has found a way to allow something meaningful to come from a heartbreaking situation.

I have witnessed firsthand Denise's truly unbelievable courage and compassion.

On many occasions, I have been asked to support grieving caregivers during the final stages of the dementia journey. Through Denise's story, I realized I could learn how to help caregivers deal with the conflicting emotions that come with loss. By sharing her journey, Denise taught me that people's grieving experiences may have many similar emotions but that every grieving experience will be unique, with different facets and pieces.

Each facet and piece needs validation and compassion. Although grief can be a confusing puzzle, the grievers themselves are not broken. They do not need to be fixed. They need to be heard and to have the freedom to feel and understand their emotions in a safe environment. Grief is an individual, scary, and unknown path that cannot and should not be pushed, blocked, or changed. The needs and pace of the griever should be honored.

As Denise says,

> When we suffer great loss, the first step is to allow ourselves to feel the pain. We excel at intellectualizing everything, telling ourselves things like "He or she is in a better place" or "We must keep busy" or "Time heals all wounds." Sometimes those proverbs can be comforting. At other times, they sound great on paper but knowing or thinking them does not make the loss less painful; it only makes us hide the pain from ourselves and from others. And bottling up pain leads to physical, emotional, and relational problems.
>
> Often when we are experiencing deep pain, we isolate ourselves from family and friends, which compounds the sadness. Instead, it is much healthier to acknowledge that the tragic situation feels horrible and that we do not know how we are going to continue.
>
> The next key step is to find someone to talk to, namely someone who will not judge, analyze, criticize, or try to fix us. Look for a person who will calmly listen and validate your feelings of pain, anger, and so on. If we do not find a safe listener, we

will risk turning into a pressure cooker with no one to loosen the lid and release some steam.

When we find good listeners, we become better listeners ourselves. During our own journeys, it is therapeutic to help others who are traveling down this lonely path we call grief. In helping others, we find that we are not alone. We meet people who are further down the road toward healing, giving us hope that it is possible to continue living. We will also meet people who are newer on this journey, reminding us of how we felt in the first few minutes, days, weeks, and months after our loss.

Keeping our loved ones' memories alive is also beneficial for the healing process. Think of what they loved to do and create memorials in their names. For example, if they loved to garden, plant some flowers in memory of them. Play their favorite music. Celebrate their birthdays, anniversaries, and other days that were special to them.

Bear in mind that we cannot compare our grief with the grief of others and that we must not minimize our loss. If we downplay our emotions, we will not be able to fully feel or acknowledge our pain and loss, and that will leave us unable to help others who are in a similar situation. Anticipated loss is just as painful as sudden loss. No one can say whether losing a newborn child is harder than losing an aging parent, or whether losing a spouse is harder than losing a sibling. Even though the deaths and the relationships we had with the people are all different, we need to know that grief is grief, pain is pain, and loss is loss.

If you are a caregiver assisting someone with dementia, you are losing your loved one a piece at a time. You will have to continually grieve each loss as it is presented: your loved one's loss of physical abilities, loss of memory (including when he or she forgets who you are), and loss of ability to carry out everyday functions. At the same time, you will be grieving the loss of your own freedom, your sleep patterns, and even your energy. The normality of your everyday life is gone and will not return to the way it was before you became a caregiver.

Additionally, you are continually facing the reality that you are caring for someone who has a disease with no cure. No matter how much you attempt to prepare mentally and emotionally for the day your loved one takes his or her last breath, when that day finally comes, you will most likely find that you were not as prepared as you thought. The grieving process may begin all over again. You will adjust to life without your loved one and assume a new role, and so will your family, as everyone tries to find his or her new place.

You may experience conflicting emotions, such as relief, regret, guilt, and sorrow. You may feel fear, anger, and bitterness and become withdrawn because you think that no one will understand or because you do not want to show or release your emotions in front of anyone. You may think you need to be strong for those around you—and to pretend that everything is ok.

What is grief? "Grief is the conflicting feelings caused by the end of or change in a familiar pattern of behavior." Thus, any changes in relationships with people, places, or events can cause the feeling we call grief. The range of emotions associated with grief varies greatly among different people and in the same person at different times.

If you are caring for someone with dementia, you are continually losing pieces of your loved one or client. Each of these specific losses can cause grief, which comes in three phases.

1. *Unfolding grief.* This grief comes as you experience many incremental losses caused by the effects of the dementia on the person. In some cases, the dementia may progress rapidly, but more often than not, the losses occur over a long period of time. Not only are you slowly losing a parent, a spouse, or a friend; you are also losing the role that you have cherished as a daughter, son, wife, husband, relative, or friend along with the relationship that you had prior to the dementia. You may have lost the spouse who took care of the household finances, or the mother who loved to shop for clothes with you, or the father with whom you would spend Sundays working on the car or a project around the house.

2. *Anticipatory grief.* A caregiver experiences anticipatory grief with every passing day, knowing that there is an inevitable death ahead. Sometimes there is deep regret stemming from the fact that no matter how well you care for your loved one or client, he or she is facing the sunset of his or her life. It is very normal to experience regret and guilt not only when you wish that this person could be relieved of his or her suffering but also when you have the expectation of someday being released from your role as the care provider.

3. *Acute grief.* It can be agonizing to watch the dying process as the body shuts down. Acute grief comes as the physical death takes place and you face the finality that your loved one is gone. A combination of guilt and relief comes from both anticipatory and acute grief. The situation is often compounded by painful emotions and the losses of the caregiver's role and sense of identity.

During a grief seminar taught by Denise, I learned about these three phases of grief from a caregiver who also attended the seminar. This wonderful and sensitive man had lost his father to Alzheimer's just two weeks earlier. He had been his father's sole care provider for several years.

He shared with us the unfolding grief he felt as he lost precious parts of his father: his father's ability to care for his own bodily needs, his father's ability to care for his own finances, and his father's role as the father to his only son. He explained that even though he knew his father was declining physically and mentally with a terminal diagnosis of Alzheimer's, he dreaded the reality that his father would soon be gone altogether. Though he had attempted to brace himself for his father's death, he nevertheless felt extreme loss and emotional pain when his father passed away.

He even felt lost himself, since his whole routine and identity abruptly changed. Without his role as caregiver and the lifestyle he had gotten used to, he was no longer sure who he was and what his purpose was. While he had been caring for his father twenty-four hours a day, seven days a week, he had become fairly isolated and had only a few remaining friends. This gentleman was very appreciative of the grief seminar, as he felt Denise understood the conflicting emotions he was experiencing. This understanding helped him to look forward and not backward.

Perceptions and Approaches

Understanding and accepting the grief process guides you through acknowledging the loss. You can then give yourself permission to feel the emotions and will be aware that grief is a normal and natural part of the human experience. Among the feelings you may experience are the following:

- After a loss you may feel uncomfortable and may be afraid to show joy because it seems to dishonor the person you have lost or because you are worried how others will perceive you if you do not behave in the way that you think they might expect you to behave.
- You might feel bad because, deep down, you are relieved that you are now finished with a very frustrating and unhappy role into which you were thrust.
- You might also feel that the caregiving was very rewarding and gave you unexpected closeness and treasured time with your loved one. Now that he or she is gone, you may feel empty.

Other people may want you to "get over it," "move on," or "be thankful that your loved one is in a better place," and they may assure you that "time heals." There will be days when you feel like avoiding contact with other people just so you will not have to hear anyone say anything trite. Outsiders believe these statements will help us work through the grief.

Denise and I and other caregivers who are experienced in the grief process understand that you would love to move on, if only you knew how. Many caregivers who share their own grief journeys candidly explain that the pain decreases but the void does not go away. One perception that may be helpful is to view the loss as a fork in the road on your journey. As you would do if you unexpectedly encountered a detour, you will find it beneficial to consult with others, look at a map, and have the right preparations to reach your destination. If you stay isolated and do not reach out to learn the tools you need to get you through the grieving process, the isolation could consume you, and this would not make the situation better.

An experienced grief counselor will help you to lean into the grief and will offer suggestions about how you can cope with the myriad complex feelings. A grief support group can also give you emotional support and the chance to interact with others who may be feeling similar emotions as they process their experiences. Getting support at this time will help you understand how to rediscover the normality of everyday life and will assist you in transitioning to your new identity and purpose. I have found that grief counseling has also proven very helpful for caregivers.

To find a certified grief recovery specialist in your area, you can email Denise Howard (deniseyhoward@gmail.com) or call the Grief Recovery Institute at 1-818-907-9600. A book on the subject of grief that I recommend is *The Grief Recovery Handbook* by John W. James and Russell Friedman.

No matter where you are in the grieving process, trust your own journey. Let yourself explore and experience everything that grieving brings you. Look for support from trusted family, friends, and professionals who will help you continue going forward.

Above all, know that you need to choose the pace and the path that are right for you. Be gentle with yourself. You are a caregiver hero, and you may find that sharing your story will help others who follow behind you on the dementia caregiving journey.

Another important perception is the understanding that hospice can be an *essential* dementia-aware support and assistance resource. A great deal of uncertainty, misinformation, and misconceptions surround hospice care and many families hesitate to discuss the option with physicians and their loved ones. I often urge families to learn and talk about this valuable resource even if it isn't needed at the moment. A lot of families just learn of the condition and are in denial about losing their loved one in six months or less.

I am a big advocate for early hospice/palliative dementia care intervention. I believe that if a family caregiver is thinking their loved one needs help, has questions, and needs guidance, then that is the time to seek out assistance. It is never too early to begin gathering information and forming a plan as a family. Hospice exists to support patients as well as their family members throughout this trying time. There are also bereavement services that are offered before and after a patient's passing. After a patient passes, bereavement can be available for up to thirteen months.

Strategies

Because those with dementia decline so gradually, family members may wait too long and not seek help until their loved ones are very close to the end. Many do not realize that assistance and specialized care may have been available much earlier. While a physician must make the official determination of life expectancy, I recommend requesting a hospice evaluation if an individual with dementia symptoms exhibits the following signs:

- Constant, elevated levels of anxiety and stress, combativeness, and/or anger;
- Complete dependence on others for assistance with activities of daily living (ADLs), such as eating, bathing, grooming, and toileting;
- Extreme difficulty or complete inability to walk without assistance;
- The ability to only speak a few intelligible words and phrases;
- Decreased appetite; and
- Significant weight loss.

"Dementia-aware" trained hospice organizations typically have specific and focused training that is designed to support everyone involved in the life of a patient affected by any cause of dementia symptoms and help all to better cope and manage the unique challenges dementia brings.

While all hospices have the ability to provide care for someone with dementia, there are providers that are trained to be "dementia-aware" and speak to the unique needs of those individuals with any cause of dementia and their caregivers.

Please check out the list of "dementia-aware" resources at the end of this book, including hospice, grief support, and grief recovery specialists. Please contact them for any additional information about your specific loved one and personal dementia journey. Or contact me at my email, help@laurawayman.com, and my website, https://www.laurawayman.com/iamdementia aware, for a more complete list of resources and additional dementia-aware support.

Scenario

Caring for my elderly sister in the last stages of Alzheimer's was the most memorable time in the life of our family and one that was filled with riches that could be found nowhere else. Now, don't get me wrong—life while caring for my sister with late-stage Alzheimer's dementia symptoms was not always easy, fun, or without challenges. I experienced moments filled with frustration, agitation, and feelings of helplessness and guilt. Mostly it was a struggle, but we, together as a family, learned to adjust and deal with it. During those four years caring for her in our home, there was very little assistance we could afford and not many organizations nearby that specialized in end-stage dementia care—and certainly were not "dementia-aware"—so almost all of the day-to-day care fell squarely on my shoulders. It became more and more challenging as she declined physically, cognitively, and emotionally and I was becoming increasingly exhausted toward the end. The only time we were able to access consistent help was when she qualified for hospice assistance in the last few months of her life.

Family members should know that hospice provides comfort, warmth, kindness, and the serenity dementia patients need. Emotions remain within the dementia patient long after other aspects of that person are lost. Hospice responds to those emotions, and the dementia patient responds in turn. Ensuring a peaceful environment and a dignified death is what hospice does best for dementia patients. To make intelligent decisions, families need to understand that many of the causes of dementia are terminal and that patients with advanced dementia are at the end of life. Caregivers need to decide how the patient wants to be treated in end-stage disease and what additional challenges to expect, such as eating problems and recurring infections. Once they understand, the family needs to decide what the patient would want for their care—uncomfortable, aggressive interventions or comfort care where they mostly get treatments that will keep them comfortable.

If the family is not supportive of hospice, it is often difficult for the dementia patient to adjust. It can be hard for the individual who is confused with dementia to understand and process what is going on and what hospice is all about. The concept of hospice is voluntary cooperation and adjustment toward death.

The Successful Dementia-Aware Approach

Hospice proved to be a wonderful service that provided a team dementia-aware care approach for my sister who was experiencing the end stages of Alzheimer's, a terminal disease. They provided this support in our home (they also can do so in a care facility or in a special hospice facility). This specially trained dementia-aware hospice team provided vital support and assistance in the physical care, emotional needs, and the spiritual needs of not just my sister but also myself, our entire family, and many of our close friends. Their services were often flexible in order to best help fill the needs of everyone involved.

Hospice companies benefit from becoming more dementia-aware and recognizing the unique end-of-life challenges that these terminal causes of dementia symptoms bring. Hospice organizations used to say that to qualify a loved one for hospice you only needed a doctor to say that the loved one had only six months to live. The problem with Alzheimer disease, or many of the other causes of dementia, is that it is impossible to say how long someone has to live, as the disease goes at different rates for each person, and there are too many factors involved to predict how long someone has to live with the disease. Medicare also wanted to qualify the "six-month rule" more with those with Alzheimer's and related diseases. The general hope is that new, more "dementia-aware" guidelines would also make it easier to qualify those in the end stages of Alzheimer disease. Doctors have also been uncomfortable saying that a person with Alzheimer's or related diseases has only "X" amount of time to live and the hope is that, with a new set of guidelines and a deeper sense of the uniqueness of dementia, doctors will recommend hospice care more often for those in the end stages of Alzheimer disease or the many other related causes.

It is definitely worth having hospice help in the last leg of this unpredictable journey of dementia care. The thing is that no one should ever have to go through the last months/days alone. So many times, a caregiver feels as if they went through much of the care by themselves. For a caregiver to go through the very end alone and without essential hospice support and assistance is not necessary—and definitely not "dementia-aware."

I have to admit, at first, I was resistant to believing that my sister would benefit from hospice and calling them in was a difficult step. I did not want to admit she was on the last leg of her unique dementia journey and wondered if this admission was like giving up on her. But after hospice started, I realized I should have asked for their help months earlier.

Poetry, music, literature, and art can inspire us and soothe us as we grieve and as we cherish the lives of those we have lost. This excerpt from the song "Celebrate the Children," by Alan Pedersen, is one example that I treasure.

We got to know the magic of their smiles, if only for a while,
Wasn't it beautiful?
They taught us how to love so deep, feel so complete,
Wasn't it wonderful?
Even if we knew that it would end,
If we had the chance we'd do it all again.

They left so many gifts behind for each of us to find,
It's magical!
They're with us every day, give help along the way,
It's spiritual!
They're part of everything we say and do,
We're better people now because of them, it's true.

CHAPTER TWENTY-ONE

Lessons, Perceptions, and Approaches

A Reader's Guide

The dementia disease process will continually throw you curve balls. It never rests. As you encounter new challenges, the chapters in this book may take on a different meaning. Because every dementia journey is unique, you will need to remain adaptable throughout the entire experience. You may need to reread chapters in this book as you gain new insights over the course of your journey.

I wrote this book to help shift the process of caring for the person who has dementia from a burden into a meaningful experience. Whether you are an at-home family caregiver, a professional, or a family member or friend who is deeply involved in the care of someone who is residing in assisted living or in a skilled nursing home, you can use this book as a reference throughout the caregiving journey.

This final chapter summarizes the lessons, perceptions, and approaches offered by the stories in each of the previous chapters. The summaries may serve as reminders; you may also want to turn (or return) to a chapter that shares suggestions that may be particularly meaningful or helpful right now.

Chapter 1. Introduction: Navigating the Journey

You are the most important person in the caregiving process, and if you do not take care of yourself, you will not be able to provide care for your loved one or client. Sometimes you can only see one part of the dementia "elephant," but with an open mind, you can continually "feel your way" through the caregiving process. I encourage you to access resources so that you can find the support you need. Every day, successful caregiving hinges on communicating with the person who has dementia. This chapter introduces the affirmative response method of communication, which will allow you to bridge the gap between you and the person with dementia.

Chapter 2. Peggy: The Ultimate Toll

Peggy's story is a poignant reminder of how caregivers strive to care for their loved ones on their own and often refuse to ask for help, even at the expense of their own lives.

Lessons learned. By taking care of yourself, you will give yourself the health and energy needed to take care of your loved one or client.

Perceptions and approaches. Adults with dementia base much of their communication on emotions. Listen to them carefully and speak from your heart.

Chapter 3. Deborah: A Daughter's Journey

Denial can make dementia more difficult to treat and can have consequences on overall quality of life—for both the person with dementia and you, the caregiver. Because no one wants to watch loved ones exhibit permanent and progressive loss of normal brain function, dementia caregivers are vulnerable to dementia-denial. Though this denial is based in self-protection, it ironically ends up making life more difficult for the caregiver and the person with dementia.

Lessons learned. Dementia-denial prevents people from seeking appropriate treatment and taking steps to better manage dementia symptoms. It allows abnormal behaviors to continue unchecked, with the possibility that someone may be injured. The antidote for dementia-denial is to become dementia-aware. The higher your level of knowledge about dementia early on during the care journey, the more aware and effective you will be as a caregiver. Learning to make meaningful connections in a very different way, by recognizing that dementia care needs to have a comprehensive understanding of an individual's loss and abilities, as well as competent training and practice in a personalized response across the board, thus further identifying the need for dementia-awareness—not just the dementia care staff in the long-term care setting and family caregivers providing care in the home but throughout entire communities.

Perceptions and approaches. To become a dementia-aware caregiver, you must reach out to and learn from resources in the medical community, remaining open to ongoing education about the many layers and constantly changing aspects of the dementia journey. Consider the bigger picture of how dementia dramatically affects more than just you and the one for whom you are caring. Most importantly, reach out to family, friends, and professionals for continuing support and assistance.

Chapter 4. Charles: There Is Nothing Wrong with Me

Some people with dementia will experience precisely the same kind of dementia-denial their caregivers exhibit. In both instances, the denial is coming from the understandable desire to convince ourselves that everything is fine. However, *denial in the form of anosognosia* is a far-reaching lack of awareness of impairment, causing most people not even to know they are ill. Anosognosia affects a substantial percentage of people with dementia, as well as those who have suffered strokes.

Lessons learned. Because people with dementia who also have anosognosia may be entirely unaware of their impairments, they will often react with anger and defensiveness if confronted about their condition. For instance, they may firmly insist they do not have a problem and they may resist seeking medical help. Naturally, the family member or professional caregiver who has to deal with this problem can become exasperated and depleted.

Perceptions and approaches. Whether your loved one is in simple denial or has anosognosia, the most effective caregiving strategy is one of acceptance and empathy toward the symptoms and subsequent behaviors, rather than endlessly trying (and failing) to correct and confront the person about his or her dementia. Through strategies such as using positive action statements in communication, avoiding fact- and reason-based discussions that could lead to conflict, and taking good care of yourself, you will be much more successful in caring for your loved one.

Chapter 5. Frances: What Is Dementia?

This chapter addresses fundamental questions: what is dementia, and what are its causes and effects? It also emphasizes the need for caregivers to take care of themselves.

Lessons learned. Dementia is a symptom with many possible causes, such as Alzheimer disease, Parkinson's disease, and stroke. It commonly manifests itself in behaviors like confusion, disorientation, repetitive behaviors, difficulty tracking or processing information, anxiety, fear, paranoia, and, most often, progressive short-term memory loss.

Perceptions and approaches. To understand how dementia affects people's memory, visualize the person you are caring for as a big 3D jigsaw puzzle. The dementia progressively removes pieces of the puzzle, leaving an increasingly incomplete picture.

Chapter 6. Jill: Into the Dementia Wonderland

Although your loved one or client's memories may be fading, it is still possible to share meaningful moments with him or her. The story of Jill provides a deeper understanding of the wonderland in which the person who has dementia lives.

Lessons learned. To connect with the person who has dementia, you must enter that person's world, not attempt to bring him or her into your reality. The feelings remain long after the event has been forgotten.

Perceptions and approaches. It is important to remain calm as you provide care for the person who has dementia. The affirmative response method is the key to successful communication.

Chapter 7. Natalie: Much More than Words

This candid chapter explains that communication, especially when it comes to connecting with the person with dementia, is largely composed of nonverbal signals and cues.

Lessons learned. Communicating with a person who has dementia has less to do with your words than it has to do with the feelings you project. Pay close attention to your own stress level and the nonverbal signals you send.

Perceptions and approaches. You have the power to set the tone for each day by monitoring the feelings you bring into the relationship.

Chapter 8. Vada: Past, Present, and Future

Vada's story is a revealing example of how people with dementia can become stuck in negative past memories and how these memories become part of their ongoing present-time reality.

Lessons learned. While persons with dementia may become trapped in painful memories, allowing them to share those emotions will help them to move forward and find resolution.

Perceptions and approaches. When interacting with your client or loved one, develop a trusting relationship and provide a dignified and respectful atmosphere.

Chapter 9. Joe: Communicating the Gift of Value

Joe's story is an important reminder that everyone needs a sense of purpose and self-worth. Helping promote a loved one or client's feeling of significance is an integral part of improving the caregiving relationship.

Lessons learned. The person who has dementia will try to access feelings from past memories that give him or her a sense of value, joy, and security.

Perceptions and approaches. Using the affirmative response method, reaffirm the feelings and language from the person's past as if they were happening now.

Chapter 10. Lucy and Betty: Thinking Outside the Box

Through two different stories this chapter introduces the concept of creative interventions, which are uniquely tailored techniques to foster cooperation in difficult situations.

Lessons learned. Over time, dementia affects the person's abilities. Learning about these changes allows you to have realistic expectations of what tasks the person can process and handle.

Perceptions and approaches. Practice patience. Encourage the person who has dementia to continue doing whatever he or she is still able to do. Celebrate the simplest and smallest accomplishments.

Chapter 11. Edna: You're Just Imagining Things

Unfortunately, as individuals struggle to cope with dementia, they often develop paranoia, including misperceptions or hallucinations about family members, old friends, and even strangers.

Lessons learned. Practicing new ways of reacting to these behaviors will give you the coping skills necessary to help manage them, thus giving you the key to making the person feel safe and supported.

Perceptions and approaches. No matter how outlandish the claim or accusation, listen and proceed as though you believe everything the person who has dementia is saying. Plan to take action that will give them a sense of relief. To them, the most frustrating response is for you to argue or to try to convince them that the situation is not real.

Chapter 12. Margie: If You Keep Doing What You Are Doing . . .

This chapter teaches how to apply the affirmative response method of communication through flexible approaches and creative thinking.

Lessons learned. You will never win an argument with someone who has dementia. If you are not receiving the desired affirmative response from your loved one or client, try a different approach.

Perceptions and approaches. Modify the environment, modify the behavior, and medicate as a last resort. (Always seek professional advice from the physician of the person you are caring for before making *any* changes in medication.)

Chapter 13. Harry: It's Bath Night!

The task of providing personal care, such as bathing and grooming, to the person who has dementia is frequently very difficult. This chapter presents helpful, straightforward suggestions on how to handle these challenges and how to cultivate more cooperative, peaceful interactions with care recipients.

Lessons learned. People with dementia tend to seek memories that make them feel safe and secure, but because of past memories, they may be resistant to allowing you to provide personal care.

Perceptions and approaches. With safety and comfort in mind, use an approach that may be familiar to your loved one or client through past experiences.

Chapter 14. Rose, Edith, and Samuel: One Size Does Not Fit All

This chapter is about dementia-aware social engagement activities, making connections by using positive action strategies, familiar items, and representations of nostalgia in your communication and care approach, customized to each individual.

Lessons learned. Simple tasks use many different parts of the brain. A person with loss of brain function will struggle to access what they have learned. Over time, everything they have learned, since they were babies, might disappear from their brain and they will be less likely to take part in social activities. They will need a caring support system to help them engage in meaningful social activities.

Perceptions and approaches. A person with dementia still needs a good quality of life and to participate in appropriate activities when it is in their best interest. Their perception and coordination will lessen, so they will need help making sure their living environment is safe. Learning about their past will help you to help them "contribute" to the household and let them feel useful and comfortable and help to create meaningful moments.

Chapter 15. Susan: Dealing with Disruption

Dementia can devastatingly disrupt individual lives and those of entire families. Susan's story powerfully illustrates the need to access supportive community resources.

Lessons learned. Caregivers often struggle with the overwhelming juggling act of raising children, maintaining a full-time career, and providing care for aging loved ones or clients.

Perceptions and approaches. Never be afraid to ask for help. Asking for help is a necessary part of the caregiving role. Educate yourself and utilize all your options.

Chapter 16. Grace: Moving beyond Guilt

Many caregivers feel guilty because they are not able to manage all of the caregiving responsibilities on their own. Grace's story demonstrates how to escape the burden of unnecessary guilt that makes so many caregivers avoid requesting help. Asking for assistance opens the door to relief.

Lessons learned. Guilt is an extremely common emotion that prevents caregivers from acknowledging the need to take care of themselves.

Perceptions and approaches. Learning about guilt and what may be causing you to feel guilty will help you move past it.

Chapter 17. Virginia: Laughter Is Therapeutic

Sometimes the old clichés are true: laughter is wonderful medicine. Virginia's experience provides an example of how to see the humor in even the most trying situations.

Lessons learned. Laughter is one of the best stress-busters available.

Perceptions and approaches. Look for different opportunities to bring laughter into your life. This can be done daily!

Chapter 18. Maria and Andreas: In Sickness and in Health

This is a story of how a family was nearly broken apart because of dementia symptoms presented by Maria's husband Andreas. The family received much needed education and worked together to become dementia-aware. With a newfound sense of commitment, practice, courage, and changes in communication strategies, they were reunited and enjoyed many meaningful moments.

Lessons Learned. It's important to become dementia-aware and realize that dementia is not only about memory loss, but even more importantly, it is about extensive and deep losses of the ability to process normal and customary functional data, often resulting in displays of frustration, signs of paranoia, irritability, anger, and aggressive or even abusive behaviors.

Perceptions and approaches. There is hope in that you can have meaningful moments, purposeful interactions, and still manage to keep your family intact (although recognizing all relationships will be forever changed). As you become more dementia-aware, you learn to take time for yourself and seek help all along the journey.

Chapter 19. Beatrice and Henry: The Power of Gratitude

Having a sense of gratitude in a caregiving role is challenging but essential. Gratitude can help make the entire caregiving journey far more fulfilling.

Lessons learned. By changing your perspective and focusing on the positive instead of the negative, you will be able to see things more clearly and better understand the importance of the moments shared with others.

Perceptions and approaches. Take the time to keep a journal of the good things and experiences you have in your life, no matter how small they may seem at the time.

Chapter 20. Sean: The Puzzling Pieces of Grief

When we experience a tragedy, grief will inevitably follow. As we care for someone with dementia, we experience grief in multiple stages.

Lessons learned. If you are caring for someone with dementia, you are slowly losing pieces of your loved one as the disease progresses. It is normal and natural to experience grief every time these losses occur. In spite of the grief, you are not broken and you do not need to be fixed.

Perceptions and approaches. Through every phase of the grieving process, it is important to let yourself feel the pain and conflicting emotions. Find someone who will listen to you without criticizing you. You must allow yourself to travel down your own unique grieving path.

The Dementia-Aware Guide to Caregiving

Practice putting these newfound lessons to use with this dementia-aware guide, which follows this chapter.

Caregivers from all walks of life, professions, and backgrounds need others to support them throughout the process of caring for a person with dementia. In America, there are millions of caregivers like you who face the difficult job of caring for an adult with cognitive impairment. My goal is to extend my supportive hands through this book and remind you that you are not alone. Keep this book close by in the coming days and months so you can find the information most relevant to your situation on a daily or hourly basis. You might also want to pass this book along to others who may be entering into the caregiving journey.

I am here to support you, and if you wish to contact me, you can email me directly at help@laurawayman.com or visit my website at https://www.laurawayman.com. Although caregiving can often be a thankless behind-the-scenes job, you are of great value. I honor and admire you, and I look forward to hearing from you. Join me in my campaign to make the world dementia-aware, #IAmDementiaAware.

The Dementia-Aware Guide to Caregiving

Congratulations! You are now well on the road toward becoming a dementia-aware caregiver. Every dementia care journey is unique—and you can also expect that the landscape will be constantly changing. Whether you are a family caregiver or a professional caregiver, it is important to remain adaptable with your care approach so you can successfully manage the dementia-related symptoms and behaviors in the moment.

Even with all of the lessons offered in this book, you may still have reservations about how to be a dementia-aware caregiver on a day-to-day basis. While it is important to individualize care approaches to the singular circumstances presented, there are many common challenges associated with dementia. To support you with caring for your loved one, client, or resident, this "Dementia-Aware Guide to Caregiving" is a quick reference tool for responding to difficult behaviors, as well as a way to practice this essential change in your care approach. As you read the examples below, begin to evaluate each challenge and consider options to put into practice for your individualized dementia-aware care approach. Then as you read the successful dementia-aware care approaches these caregivers chose, reflect on whether your care approach choice was similar. You can even go a step further and think of other options, or a combination of options, that might also provide successful care outcomes.

Here is a "dementia reality mantra" that is useful to many people: "*I cannot stop, change, or fix the dementia symptoms or behaviors. Instead, I can only manage them.*" As you begin each day in your caregiving role, it is valuable to be mindful of this mantra. You may even want to recite it out loud.

Practice and use the tools in this "Dementia-Aware Guide to Caregiving" so you may enjoy more positive and loving care outcomes. I want to take this opportunity to remind you that you are doing a great job! Keep up the good work! You make a difference!

Challenges with Personal Hygiene

Getting dressed, taking a shower, and brushing teeth can be very complex tasks for a person living with dementia because of the many steps involved. For individuals with dementia, this process is laden with too much information. Another obstacle is that some people with dementia may have an altered sense of hot and cold, since the disease has damaged the region of their brains that controls their internal thermostats. They may even feel abnormal sensations from the water itself. This adds another layer of complexity to bathing and showering. All of these factors make maintaining personal hygiene a significant obstacle for some caregivers.

Strategies

- Offer the person limited choices and do not ask questions. For example, you can say "It is time to take a bath" or "Come with me."
- Break down the tasks into simple steps and calmly and patiently explain each step, using easy-to-understand directions and respectful, affirming language. "Lift up your arms." "Let's put on this shirt." "You look nice!"
- Encourage the person to do as much as possible on his or her own, whether brushing teeth or using soap and a washcloth.
- Lay out the soap, washcloth, towel, and clean clothes in se-

quence so the person with dementia can participate in each step in the task.

- When assisting with showering or bathing, use reassuring language like "This water feels good." Let the person touch the water before getting into the bath or shower. Sometimes gently pouring water over the person's hands will help him or her relax. Or start with a basic "foot soak" and work your way up.

- Honor the person's sense of modesty—use a towel to cover sensitive areas while you assist with the washing of arms, legs, and back, or allow the person to remain partially dressed during the process.

- Accept that there will be good days and bad days. If you are encountering extreme resistance that could escalate into a worse situation, let the task go. Try again when the person appears calmer and more receptive, perhaps the next morning or before bed.

A dementia-aware caregiver will evaluate what the person is feeling.

➤ Listen to what the person is saying—not just the words, but observe his or her facial expressions and actions.

➤ Smile, breathe, and relax—your calmness will comfort the person and reduce agitation.

Scenario

"I just took a shower this morning! I am not dirty!" Harvey would insist to his wife, Sara, whenever she would ask him to take a shower. This dialogue would go on and on, spiraling into a full-blown argument as Sara attempted to reason with her once-fastidious husband, telling him he had not showered in many days and trying to convince him that his hair was dirty and his clothes smelly and stained. Asking Harvey to make these choices and process the truth about his unhygienic condition was cognitively overwhelming and only persisted in making this undertaking miserable for both of them.

The Successful Dementia-Aware Approach

Sara decided to try changing her care approach. Instead of asking Harvey if he wanted to take a shower, or giving him options about when he needed to shower as she had in the past, she instead just led him to the bathroom that she had prepared in advance, making him less apprehensive and resistant. The idea is not to do a surprise attack but instead to minimize hesitation caused by "information overload." Sara learned that when she "thinks" for Harvey and remains calm, confident, and in the moment, he has less time to resist and feel anxious about what the showering event is all about. She also chooses her battles and changes her strategies according to how Harvey is feeling. Harvey still resists sometimes even with the transformed care approach, and on those days, Sara chooses to use her time for other tasks and let this one go until later, or even to wait a day or two.

The Frustration of Negative Responses

One of the most common frustrations among caregivers is the propensity for people with dementia to say, "No!" Caregivers cannot understand why their loved ones so often refuse to do the very things they have done willingly and eagerly in the past. The reasons are actually pretty straightforward. Dementia impacts memory, processing information, reasoning, and language, so it is difficult for individuals with dementia to understand what others ask of them. They also often lose their ability to express what they are feeling, and the outward behavior becomes a means of communication. If they feel reluctant, afraid, or confused, they react exactly how most people would in situations that make them feel uncomfortable: "No—go away!" And if the caregiver inadvertently continues to share too much information, the behavior may escalate from saying "No" to saying mean, inappropriate, or even hurtful things.

Strategies

- Respond to the emotion, not the behavior, and attempt to direct the individual toward feelings of calmness. For example, if the person appears nervous and refuses to come with you, do not directly attempt to change his or her mind. Instead, you can say things like "It's such a beautiful day today" or "It's been a long time since the weather has been this nice—we should go outside and enjoy it."
- Avoid trying to reason with your loved one and do not attempt to explain the request in detail, since he or she may not be able to follow lengthy explanations.
- Share less information. Phrase your instructions in the form of gentle directive statements, rather than questions, options, or facts and figures (such as how many days it's been since you last took a walk).
- Instead of asking the person if she or he wants to go for a drive in the country, simply say: "Let's go for a drive."

A dementia-aware caregiver chooses the battle and changes the strategy as needed.

➤ Do not try to correct behaviors that do not pose an immediate safety issue to you or the person with dementia.
➤ While remaining calm and providing reassurance, redirect the person with dementia by taking his or her attention off the situation that is causing anxiety.
➤ Remain fluid and flexible, adjusting to the person's behaviors as needed.

Scenario

David was a loving and dedicated caregiver for his wife, Mabel. They had enjoyed a devoted married life together for sixty years, rarely ever being away from each other for more than a day or two. Seven years ago, Mabel was diagnosed with Alzheimer disease after her dementia symptoms worsened for several years. For most of her life, Mabel was a soft-spoken and polite lady, and David had often expressed admiration for how she always seemed to know the right thing to say. That is why it was so disheartening when Mabel began at first responding with a resounding "No" when asked most questions, then progressed to cursing under her breath, and later started hurling a host of swear words that surprised all who knew her. This was most evident, and getting steadily worse, when David would ask if she was hungry. The reaction would be even more heightened if he tacked on more complex options, such as what she wanted for dinner, if she wanted to go out to one of her favorite restaurants, and what time she would like eat. As the questions continued, she would become more and more agitated, and the "sailor talk" would progress to mean, hurtful, and inappropriate rages at David in private and out in public. David would apologize for her, but he remained confused about her reaction. "I am gentle and don't deny her anything. I just want to ask her what she wants. She makes up things and says the most horrible things to me—words I never knew she had ever heard!"

The Successful Dementia-Aware Approach

David attended one of my trainings and listened intently about addressing the underlying emotions, reacting with calm indifference to the behavior, and practicing less talking and more doing. The trigger for Mabel's fearful, angry, and anxious feelings was his unrealistic expectation that she could still process his questions or other details about dinner: restaurants, time to eat, where to eat, what to eat, getting in and out of the car, reading a menu, and so on. This information, familiar to her in the past, now just made her feel nervous, agitated, and put on the spot about giving the "correct" response. David realized that it was much kinder and calming for them both if he simply chose to give her only the information she could manage in the moment. He also recognized that going out to a restaurant was far too overwhelming; Mabel was much more at ease just having her meal placed in front of her without the before-meal discussions, requests for her input, or conversations concerning her feelings.

Refusing to Go to the Doctor

No one wants to hear that he or she has dementia. It can take supportiveness, tact, and creativity to encourage someone to have a physician check out worrisome symptoms. Understandably, such evaluations tend to produce anxiety. Additionally, people with dementia—and possibly suffering from denial in the form of anosognosia—may not be aware of the loss of normal brain function. Because they feel fine, they can't imagine why they would need to see a physician.

Strategies

- To "sell" the doctor's visit to the individual with dementia, use another health complaint (e.g., arthritis or a heart check) as a reason for making a doctor's appointment.
- Another option is to make it *your* issue, rather than his or her issue. Explain that you want to talk to the doctor about your own recent memory challenges and would like your loved one to come with you for support.
- Solicit the help of a trusted "third party," someone other than a family member, to suggest, for example, that regular checkups are important for everyone.
- Call or email the doctor in advance of a routine checkup to express concerns and ask about a dementia screening.
- Provide the doctor's office with a list of symptoms and changes you have observed (dates and times of incidents) to indicate a pattern. This way, you will not have to share these details in front of the person during the visit.
- Keep it positive. Do not focus on the person's deficits but rather on his or her retained skills and strengths.
- Acknowledge fear or other emotions: "It's not pleasant to think

about, and I can only imagine how this makes you feel. Let's find out what is going on together."

- Just be there—your presence can be very calming and comforting, such as an arm around the shoulder or holding hands.

A dementia-aware caregiver does not attempt to win an argument with someone who has dementia.

➢ Do not expect the person with dementia to comply with a doctor's orders, prescriptions, or recommended care options.

➢ It is kinder for you to make decisions that are in his or her best interests.

Scenario

The whispered conversations among the siblings about Dad were becoming more prevalent. The oldest daughter living nearby was the first to notice the changes in Dad, and then finally her sister and two brothers living miles away agreed they could not stay in dementia-denial any longer. Dad was mixing up his grandchildren's names, had several minor scratches and dents that became visible on his car without explanation, and showed up for a family event on the wrong day. The family sat down with Dad and insisted he go to the doctor to get checked out. Dad flatly denied there was a problem. He blamed the car damage on other "bad drivers"; he claimed the date mix-up resulted from several family members "having given him conflicting dates"; and he maintained that his confusion with names was simply a matter of the family "mishearing his responses." Reasoning or badgering from the adult children only led to more resistance, so they decided to come together and change the way they were communicating with Dad about the situation.

The Successful Dementia-Aware Approach

The family decided to try a "third-party approach." Since Dad was not willing to listen to them, they asked the pastor of Dad's church to suggest that he might want to see his doctor, as everyone over 60 should get their heart and blood sugar tested regularly. The pastor mentioned that he himself was making an appointment to check his own health. This worked like a charm, as Dad was more apt to listen to someone other than the adult children. By choosing to ask this influential and trusted nonfamily member to take the message to Dad and reassuring him it was a customary undertaking for someone his age, as well as wisely avoiding the sensitive subject concerning his self-disclaimed dementia symptoms, the mission of getting Dad to the doctor was accomplished.

Confusion and Agitation Caused by Transition Trauma

"I want to go home!" "This isn't my house!" "When are we leaving?" "Why are we here?" Wanting to go home is one of the most common reactions for people with dementia who have relocated to unfamiliar environments, such as a different home or a memory care facility. This is often referred to as *transition trauma.* Transition trauma is a term used to describe the stress that a person with dementia may experience when changing living environments. The length of time and severity of the transition trauma is quite individual and is usually temporary. It is relieved as the individual builds friendships, gains trust, and develops a sense of purpose and belonging in his or her new community.

Often, individuals in a new environment are trying to feel connected to a place where they felt safe and had more control in their lives. Instead of trying to convince people with dementia they are "home," respond to the immediate need, which is to make them feel safe and secure.

Caregivers may feel guilty over recent moves or placements of their loved ones and feel obligated to provide detailed justifications of why they made these decisions: "Remember—you had a fall and lay on the floor and got dehydrated, and the doctor said it's not safe for you to live alone anymore. So we found this place! And I know it will take some time to adjust, but this is really the best thing for you, since it's not an option to go back home." However, lengthy explanations are beyond what people with dementia can process. The likely result will be negative reactions and agitation. Inevitably things will get worse with that approach.

Strategies

- Give the person the opportunity to experience a different environment and "go out," such as to a secure courtyard at the facility or a pretty walking path in the local neighborhood.
- If the person asks specific questions—like "When are we leaving?"—try responses such as: "We can leave later—right now the traffic is terrible." "The forecast is calling for bad weather." "It's too late to leave tonight."
- Say as little as possible about the behaviors associated with the request to "go home." For example, if the person has packed all of his or her belongings in a suitcase and is demanding to leave, redirect the person by finding another activity, listening to music, or getting a snack.
- Figure out what actions and simple statements are going to make the person feel the safest in the moment, yet accept that he or she may feel the same way and want to "go home" again a little while later.
- Repeat whatever actions or statements work. If agitation increases, make a note of it so you can coach other caregivers or family members about what seems to work versus what does not.
- Talk about a special memory associated with what "home" represents to the person—a family pet, a favorite meal—then bring up relatable examples from your own life and use them to redirect the conversation. "You had a pet cat? I love cats too! Our cat had a bunch of kittens . . ."

- It may be necessary to access more assistance during the peak time the person is experiencing transition trauma. Consider hiring a caregiver from an outside agency temporarily while the person is adjusting to give the one-on-one support and companionship above and beyond what the care community's staff can provide.

A dementia-aware caregiver understands that every person wants to feel safe and comfortable.

➤ The better you know the person with dementia, the more easily you can read his or her emotions and find a way to create a sense of familiarity and security.

Scenario

Our family had opted for out-of-home placement when my grandfather's dementia symptoms had become too stressful for our grandmother to manage at home. As my grandfather's Alzheimer's progressed, he would sit and gaze quietly and for long periods out the window of the memory care facility throughout most of our visit. Then at some point during many of these visits, Grandfather would become agitated, turn his gaze to us, and say loudly with great concern: "Are you taking me home now? I am ready to go home, get me out of here!" This would be followed by extreme agitation and impatience when we would not immediately produce the car and take him home. At first, we would all freeze, not sure what to say or do. We were afraid that if we used any of our previously unsuccessful attempts to reassure him that he was "home" or that he needed to stay here due to his dementia, the result would ultimately be more anger and frustration. It was obvious that our trying to reason with or change his yearning to go home would only perpetuate his unaddressed feelings of loneliness, abandonment, and distress.

The Successful Dementia-Aware Approach

Then one day we were treated to a demonstration of a true dementia-aware care approach by one of the professional caregivers on staff. Instead of trying to talk Grandfather out of his longing to reach "home," this brilliant caregiver knew to simply skip any attempt to orient him to our reality and instead *hear* what he meant by the word "home." It was a feeling, not a place, and the caregiver knew she could help him experience these feelings of "home" right there in the moment. By directly talking to his feelings she could meet his emotional needs by saying: "Come listen to the music first. We both enjoy the music so much." Then as she confidently smiled and took Grandfather's hand, he happily followed her down the hall to the music activity without a second look our way. From that day on we changed our visits to ones that included sharing special memories that allowed him to experience more moments of comfort, security, and love.

Difficulty with New or Changing Routines

Although people with dementia typically lose recent memories, every-day routines are part of a different memory structure in the brain that tends to remain intact longer. By sticking to the same daily routines, individuals with dementia are less likely to become frustrated about trying to decide what to do next. Elements of a routine may include eating breakfast before getting dressed, sitting in the same recliner in the living room each morning and watching television, attending to personal care in the afternoon, taking a walk, having a scoop of ice cream, or taking a bath in the evening. While the order of these daily activities may seem insignificant, they provide a sense of familiarity and purpose. Caregivers have the opportunity to create stability by helping people with dementia maintain their routines.

Strategies

- If you are a family caregiver, you know your loved one's daily rituals better than anyone else, so you are in a unique position to customize and refine his or her routine to include meaningful activities. Be sure to share this individualized knowledge about your loved one's wishes as you reach out for additional help from professionals providing in-home care, assisted living / memory care, or adult day care.
- Leave recognizable furniture and artwork in the same places they have always been, unless they could pose safety hazards.
- If the person with dementia has moved to an assisted living or memory care facility, recreate the home-like environment in his or her room or apartment as closely as possible—though simplifying is the best route. If the previous environment was cluttered, choose to use the most obviously recognizable and cherished pieces (for example, that recliner chair for watching TV) and declutter as much as possible.
- Allow the person to participate in his or her routine tasks for as long as he or she is able—it may not be perfect and a given task could take three times longer, but maintaining independence promotes dignity and reduces physical strain on the caregiver.
- Adjust your expectations as the disease advances. It is up to the caregiver to decide what activities are still reasonable and safe for the individual with dementia to perform and which activities the person needs help doing.

A dementia-aware caregiver uses routine as a tool.

➤ Organizing your own day may take little conscious effort but giving structure to the day of a person with dementia may pose special challenges.

➤ By allowing the person with dementia to stick to his or her routines, you also save yourself from having to think too much about how to organize his or her day.

Scenario

When I first took on the care of my aunt, who has Parkinson's dementia, I stumbled often, having to figure out through trial and error the best ways to manage her individual dementia symptoms. One of the most crucial things I learned early on was that routine was very important to her. Even relatively small things that I considered insignificant would often still be of great consequence to her. Aunt Beverly moved into her own small house on our property, and as I spent more time caring for her, I found my caregiving role was much less stressful if I kept her things in the same place and her day on a strict routine. And this not only made my job easier, it also helped Aunt Beverly to feel more calm, safe, and confident. This was very evident on the first Christmas my aunt spent with us, when I had not yet seen how upsetting holidays may be to someone with dementia. Naturally, my other family members and I wanted to celebrate as we always had before Aunt Beverly came to stay with me, but we did not yet know how important it would be to keep changes for her to the bare minimum. The week of Christmas brought about many routine changes such as out-of-town visitors arriving at her usual bedtime or meal time, or a visit interrupting her favorite television show. There was even a change in environment, Aunt Beverly had to come the short distance to our home for the big Christmas dinner and she was completely disoriented with all of the changes in her surroundings, together with a stream of new names and faces, ongoing noise, conversation, and delayed meal times. These changes enjoyed by the other family members caused Aunt Beverly extreme anxiety and confusion that escalated to very unpleasant behaviors. She suddenly went from sweetly confused to restless and angry, demanding that all these "strangers" get out of her house. As the family members looked at her in shock, I took her hand and gently led her back across the yard to her quiet and familiar little home.

The Successful Dementia-Aware Approach

After I got Aunt Beverly back to her own house, I stayed with her until she calmed down. As I reflected on the holiday festivities that I had mistakenly thought she would enjoy I realized this dramatic change in her routine was what was making her feel overwhelmed. As a result of this episode, I now bring meals at the same time, bring her pills at the same time, and set her television to the channel of her favorite shows at the same time each day. And I always put things in the same place: her pills, remote, slippers, shoes, and so on—even if it is a holiday. As I have become more dementia-aware I have come to realize that change is difficult for Aunt Beverly and that sticking to a structured schedule meets two objectives: relieving my caregiver stress and helping her to maintain her abilities and cope with her losses.

Making a Move

As the dementia causes progressive cognitive impairment and physical decline, it often becomes necessary for individuals to receive more appropriate levels of care outside of their homes. This can be a difficult decision for family caregivers to make, but it can also be in the best interests of both the caregivers and their loved ones. Family caregivers can sometimes lose sight of the fact that the demands of full-time caregiving are more than any one person can realistically manage. The decision to move loved ones to assisted living or memory care facilities can be based on a combination of factors, such as

- The caregivers' health is being compromised (e.g., by sleep deprivation, caregivers' own physical limitations, and chronic medical conditions).
- The home environment is no longer safe or easy to navigate (e.g., because of the presence of stairs and narrow doorways).
- The individual who has dementia needs significant help with activities of daily living (eating, dressing, and personal hygiene).

- The care needs have increased significantly (e.g., as a result of incontinence, aggression, or wandering).

Strategies

- A successful move requires significant support from outside resources. Reach out to care professionals in the local community, such as a senior placement agency or the staff at an assisted living or memory care facility.
- To the degree that he or she is still able to participate in the decision-making process, the person with dementia should give input on the move. However, if anosognosia is a part of the dementia journey, it is crucial to share *less* information concerning their condition and any necessary care decisions.
- A senior placement agency or facility will complete a thorough intake and assessment, which involves meeting with you and other key family members, as well as with the person who has dementia, to evaluate his or her care needs.
- The assisted living or memory care facility should be staffed with professionals who are properly trained in dementia care and who will continue to work in collaboration with the family.
- Share your loved one's history with the facility staff, including his or her hobbies, favorite activities, likes and dislikes, passions, and pastimes. This helps the staff create an environment in which your loved one will thrive. It also empowers the staff to develop a personalized dementia-aware relationship with your loved one.

A dementia-aware caregiver prepares for the future and takes care of his or her own health, even if it means moving his or her loved one to an assisted living or memory care facility.

➢ Planning before the move will help make the transition as smooth as possible.
➢ Families that take the time to explore all their options are

better able to make an informed decision about the care setting.

➤ Placing your loved one in a facility does not minimize the importance of your caregiving role. You are simply inviting professionals to support your loved one's care needs while you continue to love and care for the person.

Scenario

I am the lone caregiver of my mother, 72, who has had Alzheimer's for the past seven years or so. My dad, who was her primary caregiver, passed away two years ago. Soon after I moved in to take over the caregiving role, I realized what an undertaking he had endured as the dementia worsened. They were married for fifty-two blissful years, and for most of those years they enjoyed reasonable health. Now, two years after I took over the caregiving role, Mom has declined significantly in her dementia. Her symptoms have gone beyond what I can take care of. I always feel so guilty when making care decisions for her, yet she is completely unable to make them for herself. She does not want to move out of her home and she wants me out of the house, as she feels she is perfectly able to care for herself. Unfortunately, due to the overwhelming stress of caring for Mom, I have lost twenty-five pounds and I look like I am the sick one. I have to constantly find ways of going around her resistance to get things done. I feel so frustrated and guilty that I needed to hire a professional in-home caregiver to sit with her while I run errands for three hours a day, and then all my mom does is complain that she doesn't need or want anyone in her home. I would love to access more in-home help and keep Mom in her home longer, but financially this is not feasible—nor would Mom go along with this approach, so there would be ongoing heated arguments. I love her so much but she is telling everyone in the world she does not want or need me here in spite of the lengths I have gone to help her.

And I feel so guilty that at one time, before the dementia changed her, I had promised I would care for her in her home if Dad could not. I just did not understand that when I made that promise her dementia would later force me to amend such a naive yet heartfelt pledge.

The Successful Dementia-Aware Approach

After taking a step back and assessing Mom's mushrooming needs, as well as considering my own diminished health, I have come to the painful conclusion that, first, Mom's care has become too demanding for me to appropriately handle, and, second, it is not safe for her in the house as it is currently set up. To adequately keep her safe in her home now I would at the very least need to install special shower temperature controls, offer constant supervision when she is using the stairs, put together a danger-free kitchen, install keypad door locks, and provide nighttime awake care. Therefore, I feel it is important to access out-of-home care before it is too late or we are faced with a crisis such as a fall or her wandering off and getting lost. It's all so complicated—but I realize this will make us both better, and I do this out of love and concern. I will find her a memory care community that will partner with me to deliver the care, the love, the safe environment, and dignity she deserves.

By becoming increasingly dementia-aware you will experience more meaningful moments with your loved one and feel more confident and empowered in your individual care role. In the course of this journey you will develop a deeper understanding of the impact dementia has on individuals, their families, organizations, neighborhoods, and the world.

Dementia-Aware Resource List

This is a small sampling from my ever-growing list of dementia-aware community and organizational resources. This list continues to grow and change as I continue to have the honor of raising "dementia-awareness" worldwide! For an updated list, visit https://www.laura wayman.com/iamdementiaaware.

Caregiver Grief and Loss
- Suncrest Hospice: https://www.suncrestcare.com
- Grief Recovery Institute: https://www.griefrecoverymethod.com
- Alzheimer's Association Grief and Loss as Alzheimer's Progresses: https://www.alz.org/help-support/caregiving /caregiver-health/grief-loss-as-alzheimers-progresses

Dementia-Aware Safe Space Communities and Organizations
- The Reutlinger Community, Danville, California: http://www .rcjl.org
- Aegis Senior Living, California, Washington, Nevada: https:// www.aegisliving.com
- Colma, California: https://www.colma.ca.gov
- Cosumnes Fire Department, Elk Grove, California: https:// www.yourcsd.com
- Sheraton Caregivers, LLC, Westport, Connecticut: https://www .sheraton.care
- FirstLight Home Care, Roseville, California: https://www.first lighthomecare.com
- BrightStar Care, Carlsbad, California: https://www.brightstar care.com
- California Fire and Rescue Training Authority, Mather, California: http://www.fireandrescuetraining.ca.gov
- Dani Klein Modisett: info@laughteroncall.com, https://www .LaughterOnCall.com

Thank you for taking the time to read this book as we together strive to continue to raise "dementia-awareness" and better support, manage, and advocate for all people living with dementia symptoms, their professional caregivers and families, as well as entire communities. I would love to hear from you, (email me at help@laurawayman.com) if you wish to share what you have learned and enjoyed most from this book, and perhaps impart lessons and perceptions from your personal story for the next edition! An important part of becoming and spreading dementia-awareness is listening to, and supporting others, on their journey, sharing successes and challenges, along with the joys and sorrows, that come with dementia care, thus making a discernable and positive difference in the lives of others along their dementia care journey.

REFERENCES

Chapter 1, page 4: "My personal studies in this field have included excellent foundational resources . . ."

Naomi Feil, *The Validation Breakthrough: Simple Techniques for Communicating with People with "Alzheimer's Type Dementia,"* 2nd ed. (Baltimore: Health Professions Press, 2002); Nancy L. Mace and Peter V. Rabins, *The 36-Hour Day: A Family Guide to Caring for People with Alzheimer Disease, Other Dementias, and Memory Loss,* 6th ed. (Baltimore: Johns Hopkins University Press, 2017); Virginia Bell and David Troxel, *The Best Friend's Approach to Alzheimer's Care* (Baltimore: Health Professions Press, 1996).

Chapter 2, page 9: "Caring for a person with dementia is described by the National Family Caregivers Association as being three times more work . . ."

National Family Caregivers Association, "Caregiving Statistics from the National Family Caregivers Association," https://www.caring community.org/helpful-resources/models-research/national-family -caregivers-association-nfca/.

Chapter 3, page 18: Dementia-Aware Communities

Cosumnes CSD Fire Department, Elk Grove, California, https://www .yourcsd.com/101/Fire.
Colma, California, https://.www.laurawayman.com/blog/town-of -colma-becomes-a-certified-dementia-aware-safe-space.

Chapter 4, page 26: "President Wilson 'would be seized with what, to a normal person, would seem to be inexplicable outbursts of emotion.'"
Errol Morris, "The Anosognosic's Dilemma: Something Wrong but You'll Never Know What It Is" (part three of a series), *New York Times* (June 22, 2010).

Chapter 4, page 27: "Our right brain is wired to detect anomalies and new information and incorporates these into our sense of reality."
Errol Morris, "The Anosognosic's Dilemma: Something Wrong but You'll Never Know What It Is" (part four of a series), *New York Times* (June 22, 2010).

Chapter 5, page 37: "Dementia is not a specific disease. It's an overall term that describes a wide range of symptoms associated with a decline in memory or other thinking skills severe enough to reduce a person's ability."
Alzheimer's Association, "What Is Dementia?" https://www.alz.org /alzheimers-dementia/what-is-dementia.

Chapter 5, page 37: "For example, an exposure to anesthesia increases the risk of having dementia symptoms . . ."
Alex Bekker, "Cognitive Problems Following Anesthesia," *Alzheimer's Association Newsletter*, New York Chapter, 33 (Summer 2009): 53–54, http://doczz.net/doc/4589016/pdf.
Alex Bekker, Cynthia Lee, Susan de Santi, Sonya Farber, Michael Haile, and Mony J. de Leon, "Does Mild Cognitive Impairment Increase the Risk of Developing Postoperative Cognitive Dysfunction?" *American Journal of Surgery* 199, no. 6 (June 2010): 782–788, https://doi.org/10.1016/j.amjsurg.2009.07.042.

Chapter 5, page 37: "In addition, there is a difference between dementia and delirium."
Juebin Huang, "Overview of Delirium and Dementia," *Merck Manuals*, last modified December 2019, https://www.merckmanuals.com /professional/neurologic-disorders/delirium-and-dementia/overview -of-delirium-and-dementia.

Chapter 5, page 38: "According to the *Merck Manual for Healthcare Professionals* . . ."
Juebin Huang, "Overview of Delirium and Dementia," *Merck*

Manuals, last modified December 2019, https://www.merckmanuals
.com/professional/neurologic-disorders/delirium-and-dementia
/overview-of-delirium-and-dementia.

Chapter 5, page 40: "Frances may also have been experiencing Capgras
syndrome."
Named after Jean Marie Joseph Capgras, French psychiatrist,
1873–1950.

Chapter 7, page 56: "According to Albert Mehrabian . . ."
A. Mehrabian, *Silent Messages* (Belmont, CA: Wadsworth, 1981;
currently distributed by Albert Mehrabian).

Chapter 7, page 59: "According to the Family Caregiver Alliance . . ."
Family Caregiver Alliance, "Caregiver Health," https://www.caregiver
.org/caregiver-health.

Chapter 7, page 59: "For example, a 2009 study by C. M. Kipps and
others . . ."
C. M. Kipps, P. J. Nestor, J. Acosta-Cabronero, R. Arnold, and J. R.
Hodges, "Understanding Social Dysfunction in the Behavioural Vari-
ant of Frontotemporal Dementia: The Role of Emotion and Sarcasm
Processing," *Brain: A Journal of Neurology* 132, no. 3 (2009): 592–603.

Chapter 11, page 84: "HeartMath training programs, coaching, publications, licensing programs, and innovative technology may help people
live more rewarding and healthy lives—personally and professionally."
HeartMath, https://www.heartmath.com/.

Chapter 11, page 84: "Some in-home care providers and dementia care
facilities use a program called Snoezelen Therapy . . ."
Jan Hulsegge and Ad Verheul, *Snoezelen: Another World* (Chester-
field, Derbyshire: Rompa, 1988). This program is also described at
https://en.wikipedia.org/wiki/Snoezelen.

Chapter 12, page 89: "Research is showing that some relatively basic
interventions that do not involve pharmaceuticals can be used to ease
behaviors."
J. Cohen-Mansfield, A. Libin, and M. S. Marx, "Nonpharmacological
Treatment of Agitation: A Controlled Trial of Systematic Individual-

ized Intervention," *Journals of Gerontology Series A: Biological Sciences and Medical Sciences* 62 (2007): 908–917.

Chapter 13, page 97: "*Bathing without a Battle*"
Ann Louise Barrick, Joanne Rader, Beverly Hoeffer, Philip D. Sloane, and Stacey Biddle, *Bathing without a Battle: Person-Directed Care of Individuals with Dementia*, 2nd ed. (New York: Springer, 2008).

Chapter 14, page 103: " 'Life Stations' should replicate things that we see in normal, everyday life."
Rachael Wonderlin, "Why Are Life Skill Stations So Important in Dementia Care?" Designing for Dementia, March 30, 2017, http://designingfordementia.com/index.php/2017/03/30/why-are-life-skill-stations-so-important-in-dementia-care/.

Chapter 15, page 114: ". . . sixteen million Americans find themselves sandwiched between two generations . . ."
Todd C. Ratner, "Some Things to Chew On: Estate Planning Considerations for the Baby Boomer/Sandwich Generation," *Business to Business*, February 20, 2008, https://www.baconwilson.com/Articles/Some-Things-to-Chew-On-Estate-Planning-Considerations-for-the-Baby-Boomer-Sandwich-Generation.shtml.

Chapter 16, page 119: "As Dorothy Womack wrote . . ."
Dorothy Womack, "Caregiver Guilt," *Today's Caregiver*, http://www.zarcrom.com/users/yeartorem/articles/caregiverguilt.html.

Chapter 17, page 121: "I love what Laura says here about giving you 'permission to laugh.' "
Dani Klein Modisett, "How Laughter On Call Started," YouTube Video, 1:50, Laughter On Call, July 26, 2019, https://youtu.be/PHbaLvxCqyA.

Chapter 17, page 123: "As comedian Bob Newhart reportedly said . . ."
Bob Newhart, U.S. comedian and television actor (1929–) quoted in Laura Moncur's "Motivational Quotations," https://www.goodreads.com/author/quotes/3829.Bob_Newhart.

Chapter 18, page 124: ". . . frontotemporal degeneration (FTD) . . ."
Alzheimer's Association, "Frontotemporal Degeneration," https://

www.alz.org/alzheimers-dementia/what-is-dementia/types-of
-dementia/frontotemporal-dementia.

Chapter 18, page 129: "Saint Louis University Mental Status Examination, or SLUMS . . ."
    S. H. Tariq, N. Tumosa, J. T. Chibnall, M. H. Perry, 3rd., and J. E.
    Morley, "The Saint Louis University Mental Status (SLUMS)," http://
    www.midss.org/content/saint-louis-university-mental-status-slums.

Chapter 18, page 130: "To continue to 'openly share her heart, seeking
first to understand, then to be understood.'"
    Steven R. Covey, *The 7 Habits of Highly Effective People* (New York:
    Simon & Schuster, 2013), https://www.franklincovey.com/the-7
    -habits.html.

Chapter 19, page 134: "Research shows that caring for someone with
dementia . . ."
    National Family Caregivers Association, "Caregiver Statistics,"
    https://caregiveraction.org/resources/caregiver-statistics.

Chapter 20, pages 140 and 143: "Grief is the conflicting feelings . . ."
and "A book on the subject of grief . . ."
    John W. James and Russell Friedman, *The Grief Recovery Handbook:
    The Action Program for Moving beyond Death, Divorce, and Other Losses*
    (New York: HarperCollins, 1998).

Chapter 20, page 147, "Medicare also wanted to qualify the 'six-month
rule' . . ."
    Centers for Medicare and Medicaid Services, "Medicare Hospice
    Benefits," https://www.medicare.gov/Pubs/pdf/02154-medicare
    -hospice-benefits.pdf.

Chapter 20, page 147: "This excerpt from the song 'Celebrate the
Children' . . ."
    "Celebrate the Children," lyrics by Alan Pedersen, https://www
    .opentohope.com/author/apedersen/.

ABOUT THE AUTHORS

Laura Wayman

With over a decade of experience and a strong dedication to quality aging, Laura Wayman holds an associate's degree in gerontology and is a certified social services designee. Her innovative approach to the caregiving process has given her valuable insights into how caregivers can enhance and even enjoy their relationships with their loved ones or clients. During her career, she has developed the affirmative response method, an easy-to-learn, easy-to-apply communication style for connecting with the person who has dementia. As a result, she is a sought-after speaker with extensive experience in keynote addresses and breakout programs. Laura also teaches her "becoming dementia-aware" care approach and communication techniques at a local community college in Northern California. She provides in-service training for assisted living, memory care, skilled nursing, and in-home professional caregivers, as well as valuable training and outreach for community first responders on gentle and effective redirection tools and a communication approach that works. She is often invited to educate caregivers from all walks of life about how to become dementia aware, helping them to learn effective techniques, and directing them to further dementia-aware community resources.

Contributing author Alicia Murray, BA in gerontology, MA in organizational leadership, has hands-on experience in the assisted living and memory care field. She has done extensive research on the dementia caregiving industry, focusing on individualized plans that allow for all residents to experience homelike feelings of safety and security within the memory care setting. Alicia is able to identify and utilize flexible techniques with the goal of helping to maintain independence and quality of life during the progression of Alzheimer disease and related dementias. Alicia encourages her care staff to facilitate creative activities, respecting the uniqueness of each community and individual. With her engaging approach, she helps caregivers learn to take better care of themselves while continuing to provide each resident with care in ways that can be both meaningful and enjoyable.

Contributing author Denise Howard is a certified grief recovery specialist. In 2004, as a result of having lost her oldest child, Sean, in an automobile accident, she founded the Sean Sullivan Project to reach out and help bereaved families in Sacramento–Roseville, California. This project became an important grief support group in Northern California, and Denise has personally reached out to hundreds of hurting people after the loss of a child.

INDEX